Bioceramics in Endodontics

Bioceramics in Endodontics

Edited by

Viresh Chopra
Oman Dental College
Muscat, Sultanate of Oman

WILEY Blackwell

Published by John Wiley & Sons, Inc., Hoboken, New Jersey.
Published simultaneously in Canada.

For general information on our other products and services or for technical support, please contact our Customer Care Department within the United States at (800) 762-2974, outside the United States at (317) 572-3993 or fax (317) 572-4002.

Wiley also publishes its books in a variety of electronic formats. Some content that appears in print may not be available in electronic formats. For more information about Wiley products, visit our web site at www.wiley.com.

Library of Congress Cataloging-in-Publication Data applied for:

Hardback ISBN: 9781119898443

Cover Design: Wiley
Cover Image: Courtesy of Viresh Chopra

Set in 9.5/12.5pt STIXTwoText by Straive, Pondicherry, India
SKY10066416_020624

Contents

List of Contributors

Antonis Chaniotis
Private Practice Endodontics
NKUA (National Kapodistrian
University of Athens)
Zografou, Greece

Burçin Arıcan
School of Dental Medicine, Department
of Endodontics, Bahçeşehir University
Istanbul, Turkey

Ayfer Atav
Faculty of Dentistry, Department of
Endodontics, Istinye University
Istanbul, Turkey

Ajay Bajaj
Diploma in Endodontics
Universität Jaume I (UJI)
Castelló, Spain
Private Practice, Mumbai
Maharashtra, India

Aylin Baysan
Bart's London School of Medicine and
Dentistry
Queen Mary University
London, UK

Gergely Benyőcs
Private Practitioner
Precedent Dental Office
Budapest, Hungary

Calogero Bugea
Private Practice
Gallipoli, Italy

Francesca Cerutti
Private Practice
Lovere, Italy

Harneet Chopra
Adult Restorative Dentistry
Oman Dental College
Muscat, Oman

Viresh Chopra
Adult Restorative Dentistry, Oman
Dental College, Muscat, Oman
Endodontology, Oman Dental College
Muscat, Oman
Bart's London School of Medicine and
Dentistry, Queen Mary University
London, UK

Antarikshya Das
Department of Conservative Dentistry
and Endodontics, Kalinga Institute
of Dental Sciences, Kiit University
(deemed to be), Odisha, India

Maya Feghali
Private Practice, Paris, France

Marilu' Garo
Mathsly Research, Vibo Valentia, Italy

Sachin Gupta
Department of Conservative Dentistry
and Endodontics
Subharti Dental College
Meerut, UP, India

Maryam Hasnain
Private Practitioner
Birmingham, UK

Shikha Jaiswal
Department of Conservative Dentistry
and Endodontics
Subharti Dental College
Meerut, UP, India

Shahab Javanmardi
Adult Restorative Dentistry
Oman Dental College
Muscat, Oman

Padmanabh Jha
Department of Conservative
Dentistry and Endodontics
Subharti Dental College
Meerut, UP, India

Sanjay Miglani
Department of Conservative Dentistry
& Endodontics, Faculty of Dentistry
Jamia Millia Islamia (A Central
University)
New Delhi, India

Ankita Mohanty
Conservative Dentistry and
Endodontics Anew Cosmetics
Centre, Bangalore
Karnataka, India

Vineeta Nikhil
Department of Conservative Dentistry
and Endodontics
Subharti Dental College
Meerut, UP, India

Keziban Olcay
Faculty of Dentistry
Department of Endodontics
Istanbul University-Cerrahpaşa
Istanbul, Turkey

Abhishek Parolia
Department of Endodontics
University of Iowa College of
Dentistry and Dental Clinics
Iowa City, IA, USA
School of Dentistry
International Medical University
Kuala Lumpur, Malaysia

Swadheena Patro
Department of Conservative and
Endodontics, Kalinga Institute
of Dental Sciences
Kiit University (deemed to be)
Odisha, India

Ajinkya Pawar
Conservative Dentistry and
Endodontics
Nair Hospital Dental College
Mumbai, India

Garima Poddar
Diploma in Endodontics
Universität Jaume I (UJI)
Castelló, Spain
Dental Department
Shanti Memorial Hospital Pvt. Ltd.
Cuttack, Odisha, India

Abubaker Qutieshat
Adult Restorative Dentistry
Oman Dental College
Muscat, Oman

Catherine Ricci
University of Nice-Sophia Antipolis
Nice, France

Gurdeep Singh
Adult Restorative Dentistry
Oman Dental College
Muscat, Oman

Riccardo Tonini
Department of Medical and Surgery
Specialties, Radiological Sciences and
Public Health, Dental School
University of Brescia
Brescia, Italy

Foreword by Professor Nutayla Said Al Harthy

Clinicians today are challenged by rapidly evolving information related to clinical techniques and materials, making the process of critically appraising the available dental literature for focused, evidence-based, patient-centered care challenging. Dr. Viresh Chopra has yet again put together a reference textbook, further assisting clinicians interested in practicing contemporary endodontics to make informed decisions when using "Bioceramics in Clinical Endodontics."

"Bioceramics in Clinical Endodontics" provides the reader with not only the information required to have a sound understanding of the subject within today's practice of clinical endodontics. This book also includes rich illustrations and numerous clinical cases along with an accessible video clip, making it clinically focused.

Dr. Viresh Chopra and the contributors should be commended for their dedication in compiling this reference book in endodontics by covering the background and core principles in the use of bioceramics in contemporary endodontics in a clinically comprehensible and attractive format.

Professor Nutayla Said Al Harthy, BDS, PhD, MFDS RCPS (Glasg),
FDS RCPS (Glasg), FCGDent (UK)
Dean
Oman Dental College
Muscat, Sultanate of Oman

Foreword by Stephen Cohen

As a professor of endodontics, I have witnessed the rapid advancements in the field of endodontics over the years. One of the most significant contributions to this field has been the emergence of bioceramics. Bioceramics have revolutionized the way we approach endodontic procedures, providing us with a more efficient and effective means of treating our patients.

This book on bioceramics as part of clinical endodontics is a comprehensive guide that covers all aspects of this exciting field. From the history and development of bioceramics to their current clinical applications, this book provides a detailed overview of this field.

The author has expertly curated a collection of chapters that cover the various types of bioceramics, their properties, and their clinical applications. Additionally, the book includes case studies that demonstrate the successful use of bioceramics in various dental procedures.

As a professor of endodontics, I highly recommend this book to anyone interested in learning more about bioceramics. This book is an invaluable resource that provides a thorough understanding of this fascinating field, and I am confident that it will serve as an excellent reference for many years.

Stephen Cohen, MA, DDS, FICD, FACD
Diplomate, American Board of Endodontics
San Francisco, CA
USA

Preface

The first edition of this textbook includes the latest updates and recent developments in Bioceramics for clinical use in endodontics. The book provides an excellent update on the material science, characteristics, and clinical endodontic applications of bioceramics for students in graduate programs and residencies. This book presents a series of chapters focusing on the origin of dental bioceramics, their physical and mechanical properties, clinical applications, recent updates, future directions, and ideas for future research on bioceramics. In addition, clinical endodontic cases have been added to this book, which will serve as a guide to using bioceramics in various clinical scenarios that a dentist encounters in their day-to-day endodontic practice.

This book has been designed for a wide range of dental community, starting from undergraduates, postgraduates, endodontist, as well as dental practitioners who have a special love for endodontics. This is the reason why, along with didactic chapters on history and material properties, a section on clinical cases has been added to this book. In addition, this book has a companion website where the readers can enjoy videos demonstrating the use of bioceramics in various clinical cases while it is performed on patients. This will give readers a chance to apply these materials as per the protocol in their own practice using these chapters as a guide.

This book would have not been possible without the contributions from all the authors and a number of people who have worked hard on the preparation of the text. As an editor, I would like to thank Mr. Atul Ignatius David for coping with me during the entire course. I would also like to thank Ms. Rituparna Bose and Susan Engelken for their continuous follow-ups. Many thanks to the entire WILEY team for their support in bringing out this version of the book.

This book should be of interest to researchers, graduate students, postgraduates, and private dental practitioners. It should serve as a useful reference for material scientists and dentists with an interest in bioceramics and performance of the dental engineered material. We hope that the broader spectrum of this book will facilitate the exchange of information between a wide range of dental professionals and also serve as a reference for further research ideas on Bioceramics.

V. Chopra
Oman Dental College
Muscat, Sultanate of Oman
Bart's and the London School of Medicine and Dentistry
Queen Mary University
London, UK

Acknowledgments

"Real dream is not what we see in sleep but which does not allow us to sleep"

Thank you is a small word which would never completely convey the sense of gratitude and regard that I feel for each of the following people who have made *Bioceramics in Clinical Practice*, first edition, a reality.

We all start and stay in a state of rest, or of uniform motion in a right line, unless motivated, inspired, or compelled to become active by forces/people around us. Editing this book has really been an eye-opener and made me learn a lot and appreciate the presence of everyone's support around me.

First and foremost, my sincere gratitude to Prof. Dayananda Y.D. Samarawickrama for showing belief in me and motivating me to make this dream a reality. Also, I would like to thank my Dean Dr. (Prof.) Nutayla Al Harthy and Dr. (Prof.) Mohammed Ismaily for trusting in this project and supporting me in this project.

"It is not about the destination, but journey. Enjoy the process and the goal becomes easy". My sincere thanks to Dr. Aylin Baysan for making me understand this and always sending the required positive energy and force that keeps me going at all times.

I would like to take this opportunity to thank each one of my teachers who have helped me in my growth as an endodontist. With folded hands, I bow forward to my *Gurus* Dr. Himanshu Aeran, Dr. Pravin Kumar, Dr. Vineeta Nikhil, Dr. Himanshu Sharma, Dr. S. Datta Prasad, and Dr. Shibani Grover.

I would like to specially thank a few people who have played a major role in my growth as an academician and as a clinician: Dr. Anil Kohli for always blessing me with his advice; Dr. Sanjay Miglani for being my mentor and a constant source of inspiration and support in every stage; Dr. K.S. Banga for always motivating me to do better; Dr. V. Gopikrishna for always inspiring me with his wisdom and giving me one take-home message in every interaction; Dr. Vivek Hegde for always pushing me to give the best to my patients.

The actual strength of this book is the clinical contributions by eminent researchers and clinicians from across the world. I thank each one for accepting my invitation to contribute and for their kindness and generosity in sharing their knowledge and expertise.

I thank all the leading dental companies that trusted me with this project and supported me for it. Thank you, Dentsply Sirona, Produits Dentaires, Cerkamed, Zirc, FKG Dentaire, Coltène/Whaledent, Eighteeth, Woodpecker, Perfectendo, and bioMTA for their continuous support.

I would like to thank the wonderful team at *WILEY BLACKWELL* for their genuine passion and professionalism in showing the final light of the day to this dream. Thank you, Susan Engelken, Ms. Rituparna Bose, and Mr. Atul David, for all the paperwork and continuous support.

A special thanks to Sumit Dubey, Ashwani Mishra, and Pankaj Vats for being my friends and for their timely advice.

My sincere thanks to each one of the following people at the place of my work for helping me in various ways during the genesis of this edition.

Finally, I owe my exceptional gratitude to my parents for their blessings, my brother Dr. Vishal Chopra, my sister Dr. Vandana Chopra, for their timely advice, my wife Dr. Harneet Chopra, and my children Aliyah and Kabir for their unflinching support.

About the Companion Website

This book is accompanied by a companion website.

www.wiley.com/go/chopra/bioceramicsinendodontics

This website includes Videos

1

Bioceramics in Dentistry

Vineeta Nikhil, Sachin Gupta, Shikha Jaiswal, and Padmanabh Jha

Department of Conservative Dentistry and Endodontics, Subharti Dental College, Meerut, UP, India

---

CONTENTS

Bioceramics in Endodontics, First Edition. Edited by Viresh Chopra.
© 2024 John Wiley & Sons, Inc. Published 2024 by John Wiley & Sons, Inc.
Companion website: www.wiley.com/go/chopra/bioceramicsinendodontics

1.1 Introduction

Biomaterials as described by the American National Institute of Health are natural or synthetic substance(s) other than drugs that can be used for therapeutic or diagnostic medical purposes to maintain or improve the quality of life[1]. Along with biocompatibility, biological sustainability is also a very important property of any biomaterials that are intended to be used to reconstruct body function for an unspecified duration. However, materials are also required for temporary support of functions. Therefore, depending on the tissues to be replaced and function required, different types of materials are used as a biomaterial, e.g. metal, ceramic, polymer, hydrogel, or composite.

Ceramics are inorganic, non-metallic materials that are hard, brittle, heat-resistant, and corrosion-resistant. In addition to their biocompatibility, ceramics can be obtained with biostable, bioactive, or bioresorbable properties making them eligible to be used as biomaterials. Ceramic base biomaterials that are specially developed for biological applications (both medical and dental) are categorized as Bioceramics. Porous bioceramics (BC) can facilitate neo-angiogenesis and neo-osteogenesis inside their porous structure. Additionally, resorbable bioceramics get replaced by the newly formed desired tissues.

Josette Camilleri described bioceramics in endodontics as the materials that are composed of tricalcium silicate-based cement synthesized from lab-grade chemicals and that do not include aluminum in their composition [2].

1.2 History and Evolution of Bioceramics

- Portland cement that was obtained from the limestones coming from Portland got patented in 1824 [3, 4].
- According to Peltier, the use of plaster of Paris, a resorbable ceramic, was first described by Dressman in 1892 to fill the bone cavities which were later found to be filled with solid bone [5].
- In the early 1920s, the use of calcium phosphates as a stimulus to osteogenesis for bone defect repair started [6].
- Use of ceramic hydroxyapatite (HA) granules for bone defect repair was first reported in the early 1950s [7].
- In 1963, Smith worked on a ceramic bone substitute, Cerosium [8].
- In 1969, researchers found a new material called bioglass that could be easily integrated into human bone [9].
- In the 1980s, the first hydroxyapatite coated implants were marketed.
- LeGeros et al. in 1982 used calcium phosphate in restorative dental cement as a bioceramics material [10].
- In 1984, the use of bioceramics started as a root canal sealer [11].
- The first self-hardening calcium phosphate cements (CPCs) were developed in 1986 [12].
- MTA was developed in the Loma Linda University, California, and was first documented in 1993 [13, 14] as a retrograde filling and perforations repair material.
- Chevalier et al. in 1997 found that the friction between zirconia and alumina is very low.
- In 1998, "TH-Zirconia" implants were introduced.
- The United States witnessed the first commercial MTA product, ProRoot MTA (Dentsply Tulsa Dental Specialties, Johnson City, TN) in 1999.
- In 2009, Septodont, France, marketed the calcium silicate-based product "Biodentine" as a permanent bulk dentin substitute.
- Angelus was the first company to launch a paste/paste bioceramic root canal sealer (MTA-Fillapex) in 2010.
- In 2019, Bio-C® Temp, a ready-to-use bioceramic paste for intracanal dressing was developed by Angelus, Brazil.

Earlier in the 1950s, bioceramics were used in dentistry because of their inertness and good biocompatibility that had no reaction with living tissues, e.g. zirconia, alumina, and carbon. They were primarily used for the fabrication of dental implants and prosthesis. Later on, the development of bioactive ceramics, e.g. bioglass (45S5) by Hench [9], extended the scope of these bioceramic materials as they offered in vivo benefits by inducing biomineralization (i.e. formation of apatite crystal layer). Bioglass (45S5) is composed of 45% SiO_2, 24.5% CaO, and 24.5% NaO_2. The addition of 6% P_2O_5 by weight enhanced the bioactivity of the glass [15]. However, this glass material was very weak and brittle. In the 1980s, the trend changed toward using implant ceramics that react with the environment and produce newly formed bone.

This bioglass was later modified to create variants by adding magnesium, borates, etc., for improving mechanical and setting properties of bioceramics [3].

Acknowledging the bioactivity property of bioceramics and their application into dentistry as mineralizing and regenerative materials has brought enormous productive changes [16].

Bioactive materials such as sintered hydroxyapatite (HA) [17] and β-wollastonite ($CaO–SiO_2$) in an $MgO–CaO–SiO_2$ glass-based matrix [18, 19] have been developed for over the last four decades [20].

Ternary $CaO–MgO–SiO_2$ system-based glass ceramics possessed better mechanical and chemical properties and thus are suitable materials for wear resistance, biomedical, and ceramic coating applications [21–23]. The addition of fluorides of Ca and Mg to substitute Na_2O in the conventional composition ($SiO_2–CaO–Na_2O–P_2O_5$) led to the development of antibacterials and bioceramics with higher flexure strength and hardness [20]. Ion substitutions (Ca^{2+}, Mg^{2+}, and B^{3+}) decreased the coefficient of thermal expansion of the bioactive glass ceramics [19]. In addition to bioglass, calcium silicate and aluminate based bioceramics also showed the property of biomineralization.

Although the shift from older to newer formulations is quite slow, many bioceramic materials have been developed that overcome the previous drawbacks.

1.3 Classification of Bioceramics

Bioceramics are classified on the basis of their generations, interaction with tissues, structure, composition, resorbability, and uses.

1.3.1 Based on Generations

Bioceramics are divided into three generations:

1) First generation: The first generation bioceramics are inert, thus do not initiate any reaction with living tissues, e.g. zirconia and alumina. Although they are biocompatible, for the body tissue they are like a foreign body,

leading to the formation of an acellular collagen capsule which isolates them from the body tissues.

2) Second generation: In the 1980s, the trend changed toward the development of bioceramics with improved bioactivity and the second generation bioactive bioceramics were developed, e.g. calcium phosphates, glasses and ceramic glasses, and calcium silicate. These bioceramics can react with the physiological fluids forming biological-type apatite as a byproduct of said reaction; in the presence of living cells, this apatite can form new bone.

3) Third generation: The third generation bioactive, porous bioceramics were developed because of biological requirements. Only porous ceramics can fulfil physiological requirements in their use as scaffolds for cells and inducting molecules and being able to drive self-regeneration of tissues. Example: nanometric apatites, shaped in the form of pieces with interconnected and hierarchical porosity, within the micron range so that cells can perform their bone formation and regeneration tasks.

1.3.2 Based on Tissue Interaction

The fact that the reactivity of solids begins on their surface is of particular importance in the field of bioceramics because on application they remain in contact with an aqueous medium and in the presence of cells and proteins [24]. Based on different types of interactions [25, 26] shown by bioceramics, it is classified as:

1) Bioinert: These materials have a high chemical stability in vivo; thus, they do not interact and show no chemical changes when they are in contact with living tissues. They also possess high mechanical strength, e.g. alumina, zirconia, and carbon.

2) Bioactive: Bioactive bioceramics have the character of osteoconduction and the capability of chemical bonding with living bone tissue. These materials bond directly with living tissues by undergoing interfacial interactions, e.g. bioactive glasses, HA, calcium silicates, and calcium aluminates.

3) Biodegradable: These materials when in contact with living tissues either become soluble or resorb and eventually get replaced or incorporated into tissue, e.g. tricalcium phosphate, calcium phosphate, aluminum–calcium–phosphates, and calcium aluminates.

1.3.3 Based on Structure

Depending on the structure type, bioceramics are classified into:

1) Dense: Bioceramics that are available as solid bulk structures like bars, rods, or to any shape through injection molding fall in this category. Because of their nonporous nature, these bioceramics show poor vascularization and osteoinduction ability, e.g. zirconia.

2) Porous: Porous bioceramics have attracted tremendous attention with their excellent biological function and osteoinduction ability. They provide scaffolds for cells to adhere, proliferate, differentiate, and regenerate tissues. The mean size and surface area of porosity plays an important role in the growth and migration of a tissue into the bioceramic scaffolds, e.g. CaP scaffold.

1.3.4 Based on Composition

On the basis of their composition, bioceramics are classified into:

1) Calcium silicate-based: The calcium silicate-based bioceramics can be further categorized on the basis of their application:
   a) Cement: e.g. Biodentine (Septodont, France), mineral trioxide aggregate (MTA), Portland cement.
   b) Sealer: BioRoot RCS (Septodont, France), Endo-CPM-Sealer (EGO SRL, Buenos Aires, Argentina), MTA Fillapex (Angelus, Brazil), TECHBiosealer (Profident, Kielce, Poland).
2) Calcium phosphate-based bioceramics: These materials are obtainable as bone cements, paste, scaffolds, and coatings. The tricalcium phosphate has shown the property of osteogenesis during bony defect treatment, e.g. tricalcium phosphate and HA. Bioglass, a glass ceramic containing calcium and phosphate, showed bonding with the living bone with a calcium phosphate-rich layer [27].
3) Mixture of calcium silicates and calcium phosphates: EndoSequence BC Sealer (Brasseler, Savannah, GA, USA)/Total Fill, BioAggregate (Innovative Bioceramix Inc., Vancouver, Canada), Tech Biosealer, Ceramicrete (developed at Argonne National Lab, IL, USA), iRoot BP, iRoot BP plus, iRoot SP (Innovative Bioceramix Inc., Vancouver, Canada)
4) Calcium aluminate-based: These materials can set, harden, and maintain their physical and mechanical properties over time in an oral environment. They have the ability to create apatite on their surface and provide tight seal between the tooth and itself. The cements can also contribute to the healing of the dental pulp or in the tissue surrounding the root of a tooth by eluting ions to stimulate cytokines, e.g. EndoBinder, Generex, Capasio, and Quick-set.

1.3.5 Based on Resorbability

1) Nonresorbable: Alumina, zirconia, carbon, HA, and calcium phosphate cement.
2) Resorbable: β tricalcium phosphate and calcium sulfate

1.3.6   Based on Their Location-Specific Use in Endodontology

They are classified as [28]:

1) Intracoronal
   - Pulp capping materials
   - Regenerative endodontic cements
2) Intraradicular root canal sealers
   - Apical plug cements
   - Perforation repair cements
3) Extraradicular
   - Root-end filling materials
   - Perforation repair cements

1.4   Forms of Bioceramics

Bioceramics are available in different forms and phases:

- Powder or microspheres
- As a thin coating on a metal or polymer
- Porous 3D structure
- Composites with a polymer component
- Solid dense structure.

1.4.1   Alumina

Aluminum oxide (Al_2O_3) is commonly known as alumina. It is highly inert and resistant to corrosion even in a highly dynamic oral environment. Additionally, it has high wear resistance and surface finish. As an implant material, it was first used in the 1970s. It does not integrate with bone or soft tissues. Because of its hardness being higher than the other metal alloys, alumina found its main application as biomaterials in the articular surfaces of joint replacements [29].

1.4.2   Zirconia

Zirconium dioxide is commonly known as zirconia. As zirconium is a very strong metal, it is also known as "ceramic steel." The inherent properties of zirconia such as inertness, high toughness, strength, wear resistance, fatigue resistance, and biocompatibility make it suitable to be used as dental bioceramics.

Zirconia established itself as implant material in the 1960s. Compared to zirconia, partially stabilized zirconia showed superior flexural strength, fracture toughness, lower stiffness, and a superior surface [30].

1.4.3 Hydroxyapatite (HA)

HA ($Ca_{10}(PO_4)_6(OH)_2$) is a major component of human bones and teeth. It belongs to the calcium phosphate family with a calcium to phosphorus ratio of 1.67. Since most of the inorganic portion of the human bone tissue is HA, it can be effective in reconstructing human bone tissue. It is capable of integrating and supporting bone growth, without breaking down or dissolving. It has higher stability in aqueous media than other calcium phosphate ceramics within a pH range of 4.2–8.0 [31]. In the 1970s, resorbed residual ridge repair started with HA and in 1988 in North America it was declared as a successful implant material.

To fill the bone defects or spaces, HA may be used in the form of either powder, blocks, or beads. The bone filler acts as a scaffold to facilitate the formation of natural bone.

HA is also used to alter the surface properties of metals by the application of coating on its surface. Because of the poor mechanical properties, HA cannot be used for load-bearing applications.

1.4.4 Calcium Phosphate

Examples of calcium phosphate-based bioceramics used in dentistry are CPC, tricalcium phosphate, HA, and bioglass that are used as bone substitutes and also an adjunct with the dental cements [25]. CPC offers the potential for in situ molding and injectability.

Tricalcium phosphate is a biodegradable bioceramic. Tricalcium phosphate has four polymorphs; the most common ones are the α and β forms. It dissolves in physiological media and can be replaced with bone during implantation.

When the ratio of Ca/P in calcium phosphate compounds is less than 1, it becomes highly soluble and is thus unsuitable for biological implantation. It is used as a coating on metallic implants, as fillers in polymer matrices, as self-setting bone cements, as granules or as larger shaped structures.

1.4.5 Mineral Trioxide Aggregate

Dr. Torabinajed introduced MTA in 1993. MTA powder comprises 75% mixture of tricalcium silicate ($(CaO)_3SiO_2$), dicalcium silicate ($(CaO)_2SiO_2$), and tricalcium aluminate ($(CaO)_3 Al_2O_3$) 20% bismuth oxide; and 5% gypsum. This combination possesses osteoconductive, osteoinductive, and biocompatible properties. When mineral trioxide powder is mixed with water, initially calcium hydroxide and calcium silicate hydrate are formed [32]. MTA is an active biomaterial with the potential to interact with the fluids in the tissues. The pH value is 10.2 after mixing and it rises to 12.5 at three hours resulting in an alkaline environment [32].

1.4.6 Biodentine

Biodentine, a tricalcium silicate-based hydraulic cement, was developed by Septodont research group (Septodont, Saint-Maur-des-Fosses, France) as a bioactive dentin substitute material. Tricalcium silicate is the main component and the additives include calcium carbonate in the powder; calcium chloride, water-soluble polymer, and water make the liquid. Calcium chloride controls the setting time. Biodentine exhibits a higher initial rate of calcium ion release compared to other similar material types [33, 34]. This is due to the interaction of the calcium carbonate that enhances the reaction rate [35].

Hydrated calcium silicate gel and calcium hydroxide are produced because of the hydration of tricalcium silicate. The hydrated calcium silicate gel and calcium hydroxide gradually fill in the spaces between the tricalcium grains by precipitating at the surface of the particles. Biodentine continues to improve in terms of internal structure toward a denser material, with a decrease in porosity after the initial setting.

1.5 Physicochemical Properties of Bioceramics

The physiochemical properties of bioceramics govern the application and outcome of the use of bioceramic materials. The therapeutic effect of these biomaterials in aiding healing and restoring function is dependent on the chemical reactions that affect their setting, hardening in the presence of oral tissues and fluids. The biological response of the tissues is mediated through a dynamic interaction between these materials, depending on their composition, biocompatibility, and specific properties such as surface microhardness, flow, pH, flexural strength, etc. related to them. The following discussion is focused on the physiochemical properties of commercially used bioceramics commonly used in endodontics.

1.5.1 Portland Cement

Portland cement (PC) offers antibacterial activity, biocompatibility, bio-inductivity, and acceptable physical and chemical properties when used for varied applications in dentistry, particularly endodontics. The physical and chemical properties of Portland cement resemble more closely to MTA.

- PC like MTA is available as gray and white.
- **Discoloration** – Ordinary PC (gray) shows lesser discoloration compared to gray MTA. However, there is an equal lack of discoloration seen by white MTA and white PC [36].
- **Solubility** – Greater solubility is seen with MTA when compared to white PC. It also shows better washout resistance compared to MTA in different solutions [36].
- **Bioactivity** – Maturation of MTA after hydration is more structured than PC, hence the former displays better bioactivity. Calcium ion release and formation of HA crystals is seen with both gray and white PC [36].
- **Particle size** – The particle size of white ProRoot MTA is significantly smaller than white PC both before and after hydration [36].
- **Antibacterial properties** – PC shows antibacterial and antifungal properties similar to MTA against *Enterococcus faecalis*, *Micrococcus luteus*, *Staphylococcus aureus*, *Staphylococcus epidermidis*, *Pseudomonas aeruginosa*, and *Candida albicans* [[36]].
- **Sealing ability** – White and gray MTA had similar sealing abilities as a root-end filling material when checked by means of dye penetration as compared to white and gray PC. However, when checked as a perforation repair material by means of protein leakage, white PC showed better sealing ability compared to white and gray MTA [36].
- **Biocompatibility** – Cell culture studies have shown variable result per the cell type. Essentially, there has been no genotoxicity or cytotoxicity seen associated with PC similar to MTA with respect to fibroblasts. However, with respect to human bone marrow derived mesenchymal stem cells, MTA displayed greater proliferation and migration compared to PC. Biomineralization is greater with MTA compared to PC when observed at 30 and 60 days. Pulpotomy performed with PC and MTA is successful both clinically and radiographically, but the root canals showed greater obliteration with PC [36].

1.5.2 ProRoot MTA

ProRoot MTA is made of fine hydrophilic particles that set in the presence of water. It seals off pathways between the root canal system and surrounding tissues, significantly reducing bacterial migration. Its excellent compatibility with the dentinal wall allows for a predictable clinical healing response. The physical and chemical properties of ProRoot MTA are:

- **pH value**: The pH value of MTA is 10.2 after mixing and rises to 12.5 after three hours. White MTA (WMTA) displays a significantly higher pH value 60 minutes after mixing compared to Gray MTA (GMTA) [37].
- **Compressive strength**: The compressive strength of ProRoot MTA is 40 MPa at 24 hours and ~67 MPa at 21 days [36].
- **Setting time**: The recommended powder liquid ratio for MTA is 3 : 1. The setting time of gray ProRoot MTA has been reported by Torabinejad et al. as 2 hours and 45 minutes (±5 minutes). The mean setting time of MTA has been reported to be approximately 165 minutes, which is longer than the amalgams, Super EBA and IRM. GMTA has significantly higher initial and final setting times than WMTA. Islam et al. reported final setting times of 140 minutes (2 hours and 20 minutes) for WMTA and 175 minutes (2 hours and 55 minutes) for GMTA. The presence of gypsum is reported to be the reason for the extended setting time. pH-hydrated MTA products have an initial pH of 10.2, which rises to 12.5 three hours after mixing.
- **Pushout bond strength**: The retentive strength of MTA is significantly less than that of glass ionomer or zinc phosphate cement and, thus, it is not considered to be a suitable luting agent. Studies have shown that a 4-mm thickness of MTA (apical barrier) offered more resistance to displacement than a 1-mm thickness. One of the study found the push-out bond strength of MTA after 24 hours to be ~5.2 ± 0.4 MPa. The strength significantly increased to 9.0 ± 0.9 MPa after the samples were allowed to set for seven days [36].
- **Flexural strength**: Raghavendra et al. in their review reported that placement of moist cotton pellets over the setting MTA for 24 hours showed significant increase in flexural strength, i.e. ~14.27 ± 1.96 MPa [36].
- **Porosity**: The amount of porosity in mixed cement is related to the amount of water added to make a paste, entrapment of air bubbles during the mixing procedure, or the environmental acidic pH value [36].
- **Microhardness**: Less humidity, low pH values, the presence of a chelating agent, and more condensation pressure might adversely affect MTA microhardness [36].
- **Sealing ability**: The majority of the dye and fluid filtration studies suggest that MTA materials overall allow less microleakage than traditional materials when used as an apical restoration while providing equivalent protection as a zinc oxide eugenol (ZOE) preparation when used to repair furcation perforations. GMTA and WMTA are shown to provide equivocal results compared against gutta-percha when used as a root canal obturation material in microleakage studies. No significant leakage is observed when at least 3 mm of MTA remains after root-end resection. However, significantly more leakage is seen when 2 mm or less thickness of MTA remains after root-end resection [36].

- **Particle size**: The physical properties of cement might be influenced by crystal size. Smaller sized particles increase surface contact with the liquid and lead to greater early strength and ease of handling [36].

1.5.3 MTA Angelus

MTA Angelus exhibits a reduced setting time, is sold in containers that permit more controlled dispensing, and possesses the same desirable properties as traditional MTA.

- **Setting time**: The setting time of MTA Angelus is approximately 14 minutes, which is considerably less than WMTA and GMTA [38].
- **pH value**: The results on the pH and calcium ion release of MTA Angelus are conflicting. While one of the studies suggests that MTA Angelus produced a higher pH value and calcium ion release than GMTA within 168 hours after mixing while other reported that pH and calcium release is lower in MTA Angelus than in MTA. Yet another study concluded that the pH and calcium ion release between MTA and MTA Angelus is not significantly different [38].
- **Microhardness**: The microhardness of MTA Angelus has been reported to be increasing with incubation time and influenced by the technique of mixing [38].
- **Sealing ability:** Several dye leakage studies have compared the quality of the seal by MTA Angelus, zinc-free amalgam, Vitremer (a resin-modified glass ionomer cement), and Super EBA, with conflicting reports. Wang in a review reported that MTA Angelus gave the best seal against root dentin among all the tested materials. In contrast, another study found more leakage with MTA Angelus and Vitremer compared to Super EBA in apical sections. However, no significant difference could be found between MTA Angelus and Super EBA in other tooth sections. Controversy also exists between MTA Angelus and MTA. One study showed no significant difference in dye penetration between them, whereas GMTA showed less dye leakage when used as a perforation repair material in another investigation. When an internal matrix was used for MTA Angelus, it demonstrated a better seal [38].
- **Radiopacity:** MTA Angelus has also shown to have a lower radiopacity than WMTA and GMTA [38].

1.5.4 Biodentine

"Biodentine" is a calcium silicate-based product that became commercially available in 2009. The material is formulated using the MTA-based cement technology and possesses better physical and biological properties compared to other tricalcium silicate cements such as mineral trioxide aggregate (MTA) and BioAggregate.

- **Setting time:** The setting time of Biodentine according to manufacturer's instructions is 9–12 minutes. The presence of setting accelerator in Biodentine results in faster setting, thereby improving its strength and handling characteristics [36]. Grech et al. compared the setting times of Biodentine, zirconium replaced tricalcium silicate cement, and BioAggregate and concluded that Biodentine had the shortest setting time among tricalcium silicate cements (ProRoot MTA, MTA Angelus, etc.).
- **Density and porosity:** A study done by De Souza et al. compared Biodentine to other silicate-based cements, IRoot BP Plus, Ceramicrete, and ProRoot MTA using micro-CT characterization. No significant difference in porosity has been found between IRoot BP Plus, Ceramicrete, and Biodentine [39].
- **Compressive strength:** During the setting of Biodentine, the compressive strength of Biodentine increases up to 100 MPa in the first hour and 200 MPa at the 24th hour. It continues to improve with time over several days reaching 300 MPa after one month, which is comparable to the compressive strength of natural dentin, i.e. 297 MPa [36]. Biodentine had the highest compressive strength in the study when compared to other tested materials because of the low water/cement ratio used [40].
- **Flexural strength:** Flexural strength of Biodentine recorded after two hours has been found to be 34 MPa [36].
- **Microhardness:** In the study done by Grech et al. Biodentine showed superior value of microhardness when compared to BioAggregate and IRM. Goldberg et al. found the microhardness of Biodentine to be 51 Vickers Hardness Number (VHN) at two hours and 69 VHN after one month [40].
- **Radiopacity:** ISO 6876:2001 has established that 3 mm Al is the minimum radiopacity value for endodontic cements. Grech et al. studied the radiopacity of tricalcium silicate cement, BioAggregate, and Biodentine and concluded that all the materials had radiopacity values greater than 3 mm Al [40].
- **Microleakage:** Biodentine is found to be associated with high pH 12 and releases calcium and silicon ions that stimulate mineralization. This creates a mineral infiltration zone along the dentin-cement interface that imparts a better seal [40].
- **Marginal adaptation and sealing ability:** Micromechanical adhesion of Biodentine allowed excellent adaptability of Biodentine crystals to the underlying dentin. According to a study, MTA and IRM were significantly superior to Biodentine in terms of marginal adaptation when used as a root-end filling material [40].
- **Bond strength:** Hashem et al. concluded that Biodentine has low strength during the initial stages of setting, hence the application of a final overlying resin composite restoration (laminated or layered) should be delayed for more than two weeks to achieve adequate bond strength of matured Biodentine to withstand contraction forces caused by polymerization shrinkage of resin composite [40].

1.5.5 BioAggregate

BioAggregate™ is a novel material introduced for use as a root-end filling material. It is tricalcium silicate-based, free of aluminum, and uses tantalum oxide as radiopacifier. BioAggregate contains additives to enhance the material performance.

- Properties of BioAggregate

Tuna et al. assessed the long-term fracture resistance of human immature permanent teeth filled with BioAggregate, MTA, and calcium hydroxide. They suggested that BioAggregate-filled immature teeth demonstrate higher fracture resistance than the other groups at one year. Considering the long-term risk of cervical root fracture associated with immature teeth, the use of BioAggregate as a root canal filling material appears to be the most advantageous of the materials tested [41].

Saghiri et al. investigated the compressive strength of MTA, a nanomodification of white MTA and BioAggregate after its exposure to a range of environmental pH conditions during hydration. The authors concluded that the force needed for the displacement of the nanomodification of white MTA was significantly higher than for Angelus White MTA and BioAggregate. They stated that the more acidic the environmental pH, the lower is the compressive strength [42].

Hashem and Amin compared the effect of acidic environment on the dislodgement resistance of MTA and BioAggregate when used as perforation repair materials. They concluded that MTA is more influenced by acidic pH than BioAggregate [43].

- Sealing Ability and Success

El Sayed and Saeed evaluated and compared the sealing ability of BioAggregate versus amalgam, IRM, and MTA. They reported that BioAggregate has a high sealing ability. The authors considered utilizing BioAggregate as an alternative to MTA [44].

1.5.6 Ceramicrete

Ceramicrete-D is a self-setting material composed of HA powder, phosphosilicate ceramic, and cerium oxide radiopaque filler, although it may also contain bismuth oxide as a radiopacifier. The pH of the material is reported differently in two separate studies. Porter et al. in their review mentioned different pH values of Ceramicrete reported by different authors range from alkaline to acidic pH [45].

The radiopacity of Ceramicrete-D is similar to that of root dentin and fulfills the requirement of ISO 6876/2001, although it is lower than that of white ProRoot MTA [46].

The material's handling and washout resistance properties are superior to those of white ProRoot MTA. Its setting time is 150 minutes. Ceramicrete-D's compressive strength is significantly lower than that of white ProRoot MTA [46].

It has been claimed that the material has the potential for bioactivity in the presence of phosphate-containing fluids. It also has significantly better sealing ability compared to white ProRoot MTA [46].

1.5.7 Calcium-Enriched Mixture Cement

Calcium-enriched mixture (CEM) cement is a powder/liquid material.

Raghavendra et al. in their review reported the introduction of a new endodontic material by Asgary et al in 2008 to combine the superior biocompatibility of MTA with appropriate setting time (less than one hour), handling characteristics, chemical properties, and reasonable price. This newly formulated biomaterial, calcium-enriched mixture (CEM) cement, has been made using different calcium compounds [36].

1.5.7.1 Physical Properties

pH: CEM cement and white ProRoot MTA have no significant difference in pH (10.61 versus 10.71), working times (4.5 minutes versus 5 minutes), or dimensional changes (0.075 versus 0.085 mm). However, there have been significant differences between the materials' setting times, film thickness, and flow [46].

CEM cement produces an alkaline pH and releases calcium in a similar manner to white ProRoot MTA. In addition, CEM cement releases significantly higher levels of phosphate compared to PC and white ProRoot MTA during the first hour after mixing.

Radioopacity: CEM cement radiopacity is reported to be 2.227 mm Al, which is lower than that of ProRoot MTA (5.009 mm Al) and MTA – A (4.72 mm Al). CEM cement's radiopacity did not fulfill the requirement of ANSI/ADA specification numbers 57/2000 and ISO 6876/2001 each for endodontic sealing materials (3 mm Al) [46].

Particle size: The particle size of CEM cement is between 0.5 and 30 μm. The percentage of the particle size between 0.5 and 2.5 μm diameter in CEM cement is significantly higher than that in white ProRoot MTA and white PC [46].

The effect of using CH, ProRoot MTA, and CEM cement on flexural strength of bovine root dentin after 30 days showed that all tested materials significantly decreased flexural strength compared to the control [46].

Push-out bond strength of CEM cement as root-end filling material is comparable with white ProRoot MTA. Both materials showed higher resistance to displacement when the root-end preparation has been performed with ultrasonic technique rather than Er, Cr: YSGG laser [46].

1.5.7.2 Antibacterial Activity

Two separate antibacterial investigations evaluated the activity of CEM cement, gray and white ProRoot MTA, PC, and CH on *E. faecalis*, *P. aeruginosa*, *Escherichia coli*, and *S. aureus*. Results showed that both CH and CEM cement had significantly higher antibacterial activity against the microorganisms used in these studies compared to white and gray ProRoot MTA. Both white ProRoot MTA and CEM cement showed similar fungicidal activity after 24 and 48 hours of incubation with *C. albicans* [46].

1.5.7.3 Sealing Ability

When used as a root-end filling material, CEM cement showed no significant difference to white ProRoot MTA and MTA. However, all materials showed significantly lower dye leakage compared to IRM. A fluid filtration study that stored CEM cement as a root-end filling material in different media reported that when the teeth were kept in phosphate buffered saline (PBS), the samples showed significantly less leakage compared to the ones that had been stored in distilled water. There was no significant difference in microleakage when ProRoot MTA and CEM cement were compared as root end restorations in the presence of blood as a contaminant although CEM cement showed a lesser degree of microleakage in the presence of saliva [46].

1.5.8 EndoSequence Root Repair Material

EndoSequence root repair material (ERRM) has been developed as ready-to-use. These premixed bioceramic materials are recommended for perforation repair, apical surgery, apical plug, and pulp capping. The manufacturer stated that the moisture present in the dentinal tubules is adequate to allow the material to set. The physical and chemical properties are:

1.5.8.1 Setting and Working Time

The material has a working time of more than 30 minutes and approximately a four-hour setting time. The presence of moisture is required for the material to harden [38].

1.5.8.2 pH Value

The pH value of ERRM has been reported to be as high as 12.4, which is probably responsible for its antibacterial properties during the setting reaction. Hansen et al. compared the pH changes in simulated root resorption defects filled with MTA and ERRM, and concluded that intracanal placement of MTA resulted in a higher pH than with ERRM. The pH value of both ERRM and MTA treated canals declined to the levels of the negative control after a four-week incubation in saline [47].

1.5.8.3 Microhardness

A recent study showed that the microhardness values of ERRM putty and ERRM paste can be reduced in an acidic environment, and resulted in these materials having more porous and less crystalline microstructures [38].

1.5.8.4 Bioactivity

This material is bioactive because of its ability to form a HA or apatite-like layer on its surface when it comes in contact with phosphate-containing fluids. Hansen et al. compared the diffusion of hydroxyl ions for ERRM and WMTA through root dentin. They found that although both materials showed diffusion of ions through dentin, the effect is less pronounced and of shorter duration for EndoSequence than for WMTA [47].

1.5.8.5 Sealing Ability

Hirschberg et al. compared the sealing ability of MTA to the sealing ability of ERRM using a bacterial leakage model. They concluded that samples in the ERRM group leaked significantly more than samples in the MTA group. Although there are no studies so far showing the bonding strength of ERRM, the adhesion of ERRM to dentin forms tag-like structures inside the dentinal tubules that act as a micromechanical anchor to dentin [48].

1.5.8.6 Antibacterial Activity

Lovato and Sedgley investigated the antibacterial activity of ERRM against *E. faecalis*. They found that ERRM and white ProRoot MTA demonstrated similar antibacterial efficacy against clinical strains of *E. faecalis*. This research again validated earlier studies that found ERRM displayed similar in vitro biocompatibility to MTA. Additionally, another study found that the ERRM had cell viability like gray and white MTA in both set and fresh conditions [49].

1.5.9 iROOT

iRoot has been introduced in three forms:

1) iRoot SP
2) iRoot BP
3) iRoot BP Plus

These forms have been introduced for use in root filling, root repair (iRoot BP and iRoot BP plus), and root canal sealer (iRoot SP) materials. iRoot SP is an injectable, ready-to-use, insoluble, radiopaque white paste that needs moisture to initiate and complete its setting.

1.5.9.1 Physical Properties

iRoot SP shows a significantly higher bond to dentin compared with MTA Fillapex and Epiphany. The higher bond strength has been attributed to the smaller particle size, level of viscosity, and minimal shrinkage during the setting period. The smaller particle size and high level of viscosity increase the flow of the material into the dentinal tubules and other anatomic structures of the root canal space when gutta-percha is used as the root canal filling material [46].

iRoot SP provides the highest bond strength when adapted to moist root dentin wall. Placement of CH inside the root canal before using iRoot SP as a root canal sealer improves its bond strength to dentin. The results of another study have shown that using iRoot SP with gutta-percha improves resistance to fractures in simulated open apex teeth. iRoot SP showed an alkaline pH up to seven days after setting and can kill *E. faecalis* in an antibacterial investigation [46].

1.5.10 Endo-CPM

Endo-CPM sealer is an MTA-based root canal sealer that has been developed in Argentina in 2004.

1.5.10.1 Physical Properties

The addition of calcium carbonate to the material was for decreasing the pH after setting. The release of calcium ion from Endo-CPM was detected during two in vitro investigations. The sealer has an alkaline pH value and significantly higher bond strength to dentin compared with MTA Fillapex and AH Plus [46].

Another study compared the dislodgement resistance of calcium silicate-based sealers (TotalFill BC Sealer, Endo-CPM-Sealer, and BioRoot RCS) with an epoxy resin-based sealer (AH Plus) and concluded that the push-out bond strength of the investigated calcium silicate-based sealers has been lower than that of AH Plus [46].

Endo-CPM showed antibacterial activity similar to that of white ProRoot MTA and white MTA. Endo-CPM sealer has no antibacterial activity against *E. faecalis*. No significant difference was observed in the marginal adaptation of these two materials and MTA when used as apical plugs in teeth with open apices [46] (Table 1.1).

Table 1.1 Physicochemical and biological properties of bioceramic materials used in endodontics.

	Biodentine	MTA	MTA Angelus	ERRM	iRoot SP BC Sealer	MTA Fillapex	MTA Plus	Total Fill BC Sealer	EndoSequence BC Sealer
pH	11.7–12.4	9.0–12.5	7.3–9.6	7.3–8.9	10.3–11.1	9.7–10.5	8.3–11.7	11.4–12	11–12
Calcium release (mg/l)	14.7–34	9.7–24	0.8–122.3	179.6	2.5–11.3	144.4	7.7–43.4	—	—
Flow rate (mm)	—	—	—	—	26.9	31.0	—	24.83	—
Porosity (%)	6.8	30.3–38.4	28.0	—	—	—	40.3	—	—
Solubility (%)	<0.0	1.7–2.8	1.2–6.4	—	20.6	14.8–16.1	18.5	7.44	—
Radiopacity (mm AL)	3.3–4.1	7.1	5.3–6.9	—	3.8	7.0	—	6.15	3.84
Setting time (h)	0.1–0.7	6.9	0.2–5.3	>24.0	72.0–240.0	>12.0	0.9	9.6	37.15
Microhardness (VHN or KHN)	48.4–130 VHN	53.2–60.0 VHN	36.3–84.3 VHN	—	>15.0 KHN	—	—	—	—
Compressive strength (MPa)	67.1–316	60.0–101.7	53.4–81.3	41.0–43.0	—	—	32.0–47.0	—	—
Push-out bond strength (MPa)	6.47–7.64	3.0–9.4	—	—	0.8–3.4	0.2–3.0	0.98–2.3	—	3.0
Flexural strength (MPa)	34.0	10.7–14.2	—	—	—	—	—	—	—
Cell viability (%)	60.0–100.0	55.0–110.0	88.9–105.4	40.0–110.0	>90.0–100.0	35.0–95.0	>80.0	—	95.0–100.0

Source: Adapted from Wang [38].

1.6 Physicochemical Properties of Some Bioinert Bioceramics

Bioinert ceramics are biologically inert in nature when implanted into biological system and do not instigate an immediate interaction with the adjacent biological tissues.

1.6.1 Alumina (High Purity Dense Alumina/Al₂O₃)

Physical properties: Alumina as a bioceramics insert and implant offers excellent properties, such as good corrosion resistance, low wear and friction, excellent strength, and chemical inertness, which make them especially useful in the field of hard tissue engineering [50]. A few other properties of alumina include:

1) Minimum density: $3.94 \pm 0.01 \, g/cm^3$
2) Median grain size: $4.5 \, \mu m$ or less
3) High flexural strength: $300 \, MPa$
4) High Young's modulus: $380 \, GPa$
5) Pore volume: $0.1–1.4 \, cm^3/g$
6) Average pore size: $2–177 \, nm$.

Chemical properties: They have inherently low levels of reactivity compared with other materials such as polymers and metals as well as surface reactive or resorbable ceramics. In a human body, they are expected to be non-toxic, non-allergenic, and non-carcinogenic for a lifetime.

1.6.2 Zirconia

Yttria tetragonal zirconia polycrystal (Y-TZP) is the most common type of zirconia used in dentistry with its fracture toughness being twice that of alumina-based bioceramics. Y-TZP is available as presintered, partially sintered, or those that require sintering after milling and offer the following properties:

1) Density: greater than $6 \, g/m^3$
2) Porosity: less than 0.1%
3) Grain size: $0.2 \, \mu m$
4) Young's Modulus: $150–200 \, MPa$
5) Compressive strength: $>2000 \, MPa$
6) Bending strength: $900–1200 \, MPa$
7) Hardness: $1200 \, VHN$
8) Thermal conductivity: $2 \, Wm/K$
9) Thermal expansion: $11 \times 10^{-6}/K$

The overall high toughness strength, small particle size and porosity volume, resistance to heat, low thermal conductivity, and chemical inertness make this a material of choice for dental implants and prostheses [50].

1.7 Biological Properties of Bioceramics

As human bodies are known to be a complex biological system, there is every chance that some sort of response would occur when foreign materials are placed in them.

The understanding of the active interface between biomaterials and biological systems led to several important basic ideas about biocompatibility. First, the interactions at the material–tissue interface occur for both; the material elicits a response from the body and the body elicits a response from the material. The second idea is that the material–tissue interface is dynamic. Thus, the interface is changing over its lifetime. Furthermore, because the human oral conditions are always changing, any equilibrium established at a material–tissue interface is subject to change. The third idea is that reactions at the material–tissue interface are a function of the tissue where the interface is created. The fourth idea about biological–tissue interfaces is that the biomaterials are foreign bodies and biological responses to these materials are characterized by foreign body responses. Finally, the most recent idea about biocompatibility is that it is possible to customize interactions at the material–tissue interface [1].

Biological properties of bioceramics have been evaluated using criteria such as cell expression and growth, subcutaneous and intraosseous implantation, and direct contact with dental tissues in vivo.

1.7.1 Cytological Investigation of Biocompatibility

A lot of literature is available on the biocompatibility of bioceramic materials. A study evaluating the biocompatibility of alumina ceramic material histopathalogically had shown no signs of cytotoxic reaction. After a period of four weeks of implantation, fibroblast proliferation and vascular invasion were noted [51]. Also, cytotoxicity of alumina ceramics was studied in L cell line culture, which showed that they have no cytotoxicity and if implanted in bone marrow they would not be toxic to circumferential tissue [51]. Powders and particles of zirconia when tested in vitro on different cell lines of lymphocytes, monocytes, and macrophages did not induce cytotoxicity or inflammation [52]. A majority of the published in vitro studies conducted on osteoblasts, fibroblasts, lymphocytes, monocytes, and macrophages to test the biocompatibility of zirconia observed that it had no cytotoxic effect on osteoblasts [53, 54] and did not induce a pseudo-teratogenic effect, which makes it biocompatible [54].

Most of the cell studies showed good cell growth over MTA with the formation of a cell monolayer over the material [32, 55, 56]. However, Haglund et al. [57] showed that MTA was cytotoxic to both macrophages and fibroblasts. Cell studies test the cytotoxicity in vitro but cannot examine the complex interactions between materials and host. As MTA is a calcium silicate cement, its biocompatibility may be questioned. The observed biocompatibility of MTA could arise from reaction by-products. Good cell growth was demonstrated on material extracts [58–60]. MTA induced expression of inflammatory cytokines from bone cells and exhibited good cell attachment [61]. In contrast, no cytokine production was observed in one study. The lack of cytokines was accompanied by cell lysis and protein denaturing around the MTA [57]. There has been some conflicting data on the biocompatibility of gray and white MTA. Perez et al. [62] showed that white MTA was not as biocompatible as the gray version and postulated that the difference might be because of surface morphology of the materials. On the contrary, Camilleri et al. [63] showed no difference between the two variants; however, both materials exhibited reduced cell growth when allowed to set for 28 days. The biocompatibility of Portland cement was tested using a cell culture study and the material allowed complete cell confluence [64].

The available data regarding the biocompatibility of Biodentine generally is in favor of the material in terms of its lack of cytotoxicity and tissue acceptability [65]. Laurent et al. [66] were the first to show the promising biological properties of Biodentine on human fibroblast cultures. In addition, studies have demonstrated the absence of toxicity of Biodentine in human MG63 human osteoblast cells with properties comparable to that of MTA [67]. In a study performed by Zhou et al. [68], where Biodentine was compared with white MTA and glass ionomer cement using human fibroblasts, both white MTA and Biodentine were found to be less toxic compared to glass ionomer during the one- and seven-day observation period. The authors commented that despite the uneven and crystalline surface topography of both Biodentine and MTA compared to the smooth surface texture of the glass ionomer, cell adhesion and growth were determined to be more favorable in the aforementioned materials compared to glass ionomer.

Calcium phosphate bioceramics, depending on their chemical composition and physical features, may favor either stem cell proliferation or differentiation. Blocks of bioceramics presenting rough surfaces and a higher number of micro- and macro-porosity favor cell viability, proliferation, and differentiation over biomaterials with smooth surfaces and less porosity, even if their chemical composition is considered less favorable for osteogenesis [69]. Thus, it can be said that bioceramic materials in general are less cytotoxic and more biocompatible.

1.7.2 Subcutaneous and Intraosseous Implantation

Histological evaluation of tissue reaction has been evaluated by subcutaneous and intraosseous implantation of the materials in test animals.

When the histologic reaction was examined after surgical insertion of alumina ceramic in the knee joints of Japanese white rabbits, it was observed that alumina ceramic induced weak tissue reaction. When the osteointegration of zirconia was investigated in rats by means of histomorphometry, it was seen that zirconia was biocompatible in vitro [51]. In addition, Styles et al. [70] in their study concluded that when zirconia was tested in different physical forms, it did not induce cytotoxicity in soft tissues. Also, it appeared that the various forms of zirconia tested in hard tissues did not induce any adverse reaction or local toxic effects.

Subcutaneous implantation in rats showed that MTA initially elicited severe reactions with coagulation necrosis and dystrophic calcification. The reactions, however, subsided with time [71, 72]. Reactions to intraosseous implants of MTA were less intense than with subcutaneous implantation. Osteogenesis occurred in association with these implants [71]. With intraosseous implantation, the tissue reactions to the material subsided with time over a period of 12 weeks [73]. In another study, MTA was shown to be biocompatible and did not produce any adverse effect on microcirculation of the connective tissue [74]. Implantation of Portland cement in rat mandibles of guinea pigs showed that it was biocompatible [75]. Therefore, most studies have shown that the initial reaction seen after implantation of bioceramic materials subsided with time.

1.7.3 Periradicular Tissue Reactions

When MTA was used for root-end filling in vivo, less periradicular inflammation was reported compared with amalgam [76]. The presence of cementum on the surface of MTA was a frequent finding [77]. MTA induced apical hard tissue formation with significantly greater consistency, but not quantity [78]. Also, MTA supported almost complete regeneration of the periradicular periodontium when used as a root-end filling material on non-infected teeth [79]. The most characteristic tissue reaction to MTA was the presence of organizing connective tissue with occasional signs of inflammation after the first postoperative week [80]. Early tissue healing events after MTA root-end filling were characterized by hard tissue formation on the peripheral root walls along the MTA–soft tissue interface [80]. It has been seen that when either fresh or set MTA was used after apical surgery there was cementum deposition [81]. In addition, MTA showed the most favorable periapical tissue response of the three materials tested, with formation of cemental coverage over MTA [82]. Hence, most studies in vivo have shown a favorable tissue response to MTA.

It has been observed that a tricalcium phosphate compound used in a bony defect promoted osteogenesis or new bone formation. Hench [27] in 1971 developed a calcium phosphate-containing glass ceramic known as bioglass. He showed that it chemically bonded with the host bone through a calcium phosphate rich layer. Biphasic calcium phosphate (BCP) bioceramics have been considered optimum bone graft substitutes because of their proven safety, osteoconductivity, and bioactivity [69]. CaP bioceramics are considered bioactive materials because they partially dissolve in vivo by either cellular or extracellular activity or both [83]. Cellular resorption usually occurs by macrophages and osteoclasts; this active cellular process is equivalent to bone remodeling [84]. The core mechanism of bioactivity is the partial dissolution and release of ionic products in vivo, elevating the local concentrations of calcium and phosphate ions and precipitating a biological apatite on the surface of the ceramics [84].

1.7.4 Pulpal Reactions

MTA used for pulp capping or partial pulpotomy stimulates reparative dentin formation. MTA-capped pulps showed complete bridge formation with no signs of inflammation [85, 86]. Similar results were obtained when MTA was placed over pulp stumps following pulpotomy [87]. This hard tissue bridge formed over the pulp was documented after using ProRoot MTA and MTA Angelus and both gray and white Portland cement. Histological evaluation showed that both types of material were equally effective as pulp protection materials [88].

The biocompatibility of Biodentine was investigated through its direct application to human pulp cells simulating the direct pulp condition and indirectly through a dentin slice to simulate its indirect pulp capping. Under both conditions, Biodentine was not found to affect target cell viability under in vivo application conditions [66]. Additionally, when Biodentine was applied onto human pulp cells to investigate its effects on their specific functions by studying the expression of odontoblast specific functions such as expression of nestin (a human odontoblast specific marker) and dentin sialoprotein, Biodentine was found not to inhibit the expression of these proteins but rather induce their expression and the cells' mineralization capacity [66, 89, 90].

Additionally, when Biodentine was used for vital pulp therapy in vivo, investigations carried out on different animal models showed that this material induced tertiary dentin synthesis when applied as direct or indirect pulp capping material in rat teeth [91, 92]. In case of direct pulp capping, the dentin bridge formation observed after four weeks in rat teeth was tubular and its porosity was similar to that of MTA [92]. Similar results were demonstrated in miniature swine teeth. After pulp capping with Biodentine, no pulp inflammation was observed while a thick dentin bridge was formed after three and eight8 weeks [93]. This mineralization seems to be due to the release of a growth factor, namely transforming factor beta 1 (TGF-b1) from pulp cells. This factor has been shown to be involved in odontoblastic differentiation and recent investigations revealed that this factor is involved in the recruitment of pulp stem cells to TGF-b1 production site [94]. In a study by Laurent et al. [89] Biodentine was found to significantly increase TGF-b1 secretion from pulp cells. TGF is a growth factor that plays a role in angiogenesis, recruitment of progenitor cells, cell differentiation, and mineralization. Interestingly, increase in TGF-b1 was significant whatever the ratio between the Biodentine surface area and cell culture volume [89]. This is an important clinical information because it indicates that this cement can be applied onto the pulp whatever be the surface area of the injured pulp. Additionally, investigation on the application of Biodentine in pulpotomy in primary pig teeth and comparison with formacresol and white MTA suggested that Biodentine showed no inflammation and a thick dentin bridge formed in 90% of the cases, which was comparable to the results obtained with WMTA [95]. This result gives an indication about the biocompatibility of these materials and their suitability for pulp capping and pulpotomy.

A recently published article focused on the influence of Biodentine from another perspective and assessed the proliferative, migratory, and adhesion effect of different concentrations of the material on human dental pulp stem cells (hDP-SCs) obtained from impacted third molars. Results showed increased proliferation of stem cells at 0.2 and 2 mg/ml concentrations while the cellular activity decreased significantly at higher concentration of 20 mg/ml. Biodentine favorably affected healing when placed directly in contact with the pulp by enhancing the proliferation, migration, and adhesion of human dental pulp stem cells, confirming the bioactive and biocompatible characteristics of the material [96].

The dentinogenic effects of CaP materials and the formation of dentin bridge have been studied on pulp amputation and on pulp capping. Boyde and Jones [97] in 1983 had demonstrated the homogeneity of dentin formation at the surface of CaP. Energy dispersive Xray (EDX) microanalysis indicated that the newly formed mineralized tissue contained essentially Ca and P, with small amounts of Mg, as in normal dentin [98]. The principle of primary mineralization is different: the size of the particles is probably an important factor. The bridge obtained with microparticles of HA, TCP, and BCP was like a classical dentin bridge obtained with CH. Perhaps the microparticles are more easily absorbed by multinuclear giant cells or the macroparticles could promote the formation of a collagen fiber network. It is possible that microparticles are more irritative for pulpal tissue than the large particles and promote dystrophic mineralization. However, it was noticed that the microparticles formed a dense package in contact with the pulp. The bridge extended beyond the capping material with no necrotic layer using calcium phosphate materials. On the other hand, the macroparticles appeared to push in pulpal tissue, and the mineralization was formed around and in close contact with them [99].

1.7.5 Antibacterial Properties

A number of studies have investigated the antimicrobial effects of bioceramic materials. In a study that compared the inhibition of growth and adhesion of selected oral bacteria on titanium and zirconia implants, difference was found in the adhesion of some selected oral bacteria. But in an in vivo study, zirconia showed significantly lesser adhesion of bacteria than titanium [100].

Al-Hazaimi et al. [101] in 2006 stated that MTA has antibacterial effect especially against *E. faecalis* and *Streptococcus sanguis*. On the contrary, Torabinejad et al. [102] in 1995 showed that MTA had no antimicrobial action against any of the anaerobes. But it did show certain effect on facultative bacteria. In a study by Bhavana et al. [103] in 2015, Biodentine showed stronger inhibitory effect than MTA on *Streptococcus mutans*, *E. faecalis*, and *C. albicans*. Moreover, Asgary et al. [104] in 2007 found that antibacterial properties of calcium-enriched mixture (CEM) cement against *E. faecalis* were higher than those of MTA. According to Koruyucu et al. [105] in 2015, Biodentine and MTA showed similar antibacterial effects against *E. faecalis*. Also, the effect of CEM against gram-negative, gram-positive, and cocci/bacilli bacteria were compared with MTA and calcium hydroxide (CH) and the results showed comparable antibacterial effects with CH and significantly better results than MTA [58]. Recently, Esteki et al. [106] in 2021 concluded that MTA, Biodentine, and CEM had growth inhibitory effects on the microorganisms tested. However, compared with MTA, Biodentine showed greater inhibitory effects against *E. faecalis* and *C. albicans*, which are resistant microorganisms in endodontic treatment. Hence, Biodentine with its potent antimicrobial effect can be considered as an appropriate alternative to MTA and CEM cement in endodontic treatment. In another study, antibacterial activity of ERRM was compared with MTA, and the results demonstrated similar antimicrobial properties during their setting reaction against ten clinical strains of *E. faecalis* [49].

1.8 Application of Bioceramics in Dentistry

- Bioceramics have a wide array of applications in various fields of dentistry. In endodontics, bioactive BCs are frequently used in root canal obturation, perforation repair, retrograde root canal filling, apexification, and vital pulp therapy or regenerative endodontic procedures such as pulpotomies and revascularization. MTA and Biodentine have been most commonly used for the above-mentioned procedures and have produced positive treatment outcomes in both pediatric and adult patients [107]. Recently, BCs like Bio-C Temp have also been used as intracanal medicaments and have shown significant increase over time in the collagen content and in the immune expression of IL-10, a cytokine involved in the tissue repair.

- In restorative dentistry, BCs (glass ceramics) can be used as a temporary enamel substitute in Class II restorations and even as a permanent dentin substitute in large carious lesions especially in cases where the dentin is hypersensitive [108].
- Bioinert ceramics like zirconia and alumina are currently being used for improvement of aesthetics and for prosthetic rehabilitation by being included in all ceramic crowns [109], bridges and prosthesis, and prosthetic device implants or as implant coatings to improve osteointegration and biocompatibility [110]. Use of biphasic calcium phosphate BCs (composed of an intimate mixture of hydroxyapatite [HA] and β-tricalcium phosphate [β-TCP]) in the management of facial disharmony and facial deformities (caused by congenital malformations, trauma, infection, or tumors) has also shown to have good treatment outcomes [111].
- In orthodontics, bioglass particulates can be used in the form of pastes around orthodontic brackets that form a protective interaction layer on enamel surface and decrease the risk of enamel erosion by protecting against demineralization in acidic environment, and is especially useful in high caries-risk patients [112]. A combined paste of fluoride and bioactive glass pastes has been shown to further reduce the risk of eroding enamel in such cases [113].
- In periodontics, BCs can be used as periodontal regenerative material [114]. CPCs are used as bone defects filler and scaffold for bone formation that provides histocompatible healing of periodontal tissues [115]. These regenerative materials are also available as nano-hydroxyapatite (nHAP) that can be used as temporary osteoconductive grafts to aid the ingrowth of viable bone; however, these may not be intended to provide structural support. Such BCs can be used for clinical applications such as reconstructing bone defects caused by trauma, filling of periodontal defects, cystectomy filling, filling of alveolar bone defect, or during osteotomies, etc. [116]. Teeth exhibiting periodontal disease can be repaired using BCs where crushed bioglass particles (90–700 μm) are mixed with saline and placed around the tooth to stimulate bone growth 117].
- In oral and maxillofacial surgery, BCs have been used as an addition to or a substitute for autogenous bone [118] in filling surgical bone defects, joint replacements, alveolar bone augmentation, orbital floor fracture, sinus obliteration, and so on. [119, 120]. BCs in the form of porous HAP granules are very popular as bone defects fillers. HAP can be used to fill voids or defects in bones in the form of powders, porous blocks, or beads [121]. As an alternative to bone grafts, the bone filler acts as a scaffold and promotes the rapid filling of the gap by naturally forming bone [122].
  HAP is indicated for bone grafting in defects after the removal of bone cysts, augmentation of the atrophied alveolar ridge, sinus floor elevation, filling of alveolar defects following tooth extraction, filling of extraction defects to create an implant bed, defects after surgical removal of retained teeth or corrective osteotomies, and other multi-walled bone defects of the alveolar ridge [123].

- Another BC, β-TCP, is receiving growing attention as a raw material for several injectable hydraulic bone cements and composites for bone repair filling, acetabulum reconstruction, and metaphyseal fractures. These grafts are indicated for filling of small bony defects, implantology (defect augmentation, elevation of sinus floor, etc.), and grafting after cyst removal [111].
- 3D printed BC(CSi-Mg10) scaffolds are being used as an efficient alternative for bone reconstruction in maxillofacial or craniofacial conditions. They are highly recommended because of their interconnected 3D porous structure, high mechanical strength, excellent bioactivity, and adequate biodegradation, and have a rapid fabrication time of 24 hours. These porous scaffolds stimulate bone regeneration without the aid of any osteogenic factor [124].
- Metallic implants are often associated with poor osseointegration, implant-associated infections, and poor biofunctionality. To overcome these issues, metal implants can be coated with bioresorbable and bioactive BCs (HAP coated or glass ceramic coated), which not only improve their biocompatibility but also function as resorbable lattices providing a temporary framework that is dissolved with time and replaced with body tissues, thus playing a vital role in uncemented implant fixation [3].
- In oral medicine, BCs can be used as drug carriers for antitumor drugs (low molecular weight drugs, high molecular weight biomolecules, or delivery of ions). CPC-based drug carriers work by encapsulating drugs and improving their biodistribution and pharmacokinetic properties. Improvement in the specificity and accuracy of treatment can be achieved by incorporating monoclonal antibodies and receptor-specific peptides that help in targeted delivery of these drugs leading to better accumulation at tumor sites [10].

1.9 Advantages of Bioceramics

- BCs are extremely biocompatible (nontoxic) ceramic materials that are chemically stable within the biological environment and have good antibacterial and antifungal activity [2, 125].
- BCs favor the regeneration of bone tissues because of their osteoinductive, osteoconductive, and bioresorbable properties [126, 127]. They can get rapidly integrated into the human body by forming a bond to bone leading to indistinguishable unions. The intrinsic osteoinductive capacity of BCs is supported by their ability to absorb osteoinductive substances and stimulate osteoblast cells. In addition, BCs also stimulate angiogenesis (enhances the expression of vascular endothelial growth factor (VEGF) leading to rapid vascular ingrowth during new bone formation, thus playing a vital role in regeneration. BCs can

also function as a regenerative scaffold of resorbable lattices that provide a framework that is eventually dissolved as the body rebuilds tissue.

- BCs can form a chemical bond with the dentin microstructure (because of the formation of hydroxyapatite during the setting process), thus leading to an excellent fluid tight seal with dentin. This property along with its antimicrobial nature has led to its ability to be used as a bonded restoration along with several other clinical applications.

- BCs do not shrink upon setting; rather, they actually expand slightly once the setting process is completed making them dimensionally stable. This property and the chemical bonding with dentin impart an excellent sealing ability to the material.

- BCs also possess good radiopacity, which is a prerequisite for dental materials to verify their proper placement in the intended clinical application.

- These are non-immunogenic and hence do not elicit an immune reaction on coming in contact with vital tissues like pulp.

- Furthermore, in cases of overfilling during the process of obturation or procedures like perforation repair, BCs will not result in a significant inflammatory response.

- BCs possess antibacterial properties because of the phenomenon of bacterial sequestration that occurs after the precipitation of materials in situ after setting. Bacterial adhesion is prevented by the formation of porous powders containing nanocrystals (1–3 nm diameter).

- Glass ceramic prosthetics such as those fabricated with zirconia and alumina offer several advantages including ease of fabrication, high strength with low processing shrinkage, reduced damage due to abrasion and chemicals, resistance to thermal shock, and excellent polishability. Additionally, the intrinsic property of translucency imparts lifelike aesthetics to restorations [128].

1.9.1 Regenerative Endodontic Therapy

Use of BCs in regenerative endodontic therapy (RET) enhances blood clot stabilization, provides for an antibacterial and anti-inflammatory action, and stimulates tissue repair, secretion and action of BMPs, and other growth factors. BCs have the ability not only to stimulate undifferentiated stem cells to form pulp-like tissue but also induce hard tissue formation and help in providing a tight seal [2].

1.9.2 Advantages of BCs When Used as a Sealer/Obturating Material

- Hydraulic cement pastes of BCs have been developed for obturation and sealing of root canals. These sealers offer several advantages such as increased pH during setting, high antimicrobial activity, biocompatibility, and bioactivity

when set with long-term dimensional stability. In addition, they are easy to manipulate and form a good bond at the cement–dentin interface, thus providing a good sealing ability [36, 128].
- Some BC sealers like CeraSeal are also highly resistant to initial washout because of the shorter setting time [109, 111].

1.10   Limitations

Older BC materials like Portland cements (PC) have many inherent drawbacks such as releasing high amounts of lead and arsenic, higher solubility, excessive setting expansion (jeopardizing the long-term seal of the material), lower compressive strength, and reduced long-term efficacy of the material [129].

Although newer BCs have come up with improved properties, some of the issues still remain unresolved. Mineral trioxide aggregate (MTA) has good biological properties but is expensive and has a long setting time and difficulty in handling with a potential for tooth discoloration when used for restorations and in endodontics. Also, the absence of a known solvent for this material poses difficulty in its removal after placement when used in root canals in endodontics [36].

Although BCs are excellent biomaterials, there are certain drawbacks that are inherent to it being a ceramic material. BCs in general have poor mechanical properties, i.e. they have a high Young modulus and low fracture toughness (brittle in nature), which is a reason for their inferior workability [130].

Brittleness is not a problem if BCs are used in stress-free positions but their use becomes limited in positions where high stress is loaded, which makes the usage of BC unreliable in bulk form for load-bearing applications [131].

The retrievability of BCs when used as sealers for obturation also remains a clinical problem, although it has been claimed that some sealers like Bio-C can be easily removed from the root canal with the conventional gutta-percha removal techniques [118, 131].

1.11   Future Trends

- To overcome the limited mechanical properties of BCs, utilizing bioengineering technology for substitution of strong metal ions in the glass network of BCs or fabrication of BCs with hard polymer composite can help to achieve better material for restoration. However, detailed analysis of such materials would be imperative especially in terms of their structural properties, mechanical properties, and in vitro/in vivo compatibility before their actual clinical usage [132].

- The use of 3D-printed calcium silicate scaffolds and their modifications (like functionalization) can be utilized in the future as an effective method for regulating odontogenesis or regeneration of dentin or other hard tissues [124].
- Because of their low coefficient of friction for lubricating surfaces, they can find an important role in joint prosthesis (for replacement of temporomandibular joint [TMJ] joints).
- It has been seen that external and internal functionalization (coating of 3D-printed Ca-Si BC scaffolds with highly photothermal materials) renders desirable photothermal properties to BCs that enhances their antitumor potential (as seen in both in vitro and in vivo studies) [132]. This property can be utilized and explored further for antitumor therapy. In the future, development of such superior biomaterials having both antitumor properties and the potential for osteogenic repair would increase the prognosis of cancer patients, decrease their need and time for hospitalization and reduce the possibility of hospital-acquired infection [133].
- A promising use of BCs in the field of regeneration would be to combine the potential advantages of these nanostructured biomaterials with newly generated ameloblasts, odontoblasts, cementoblasts, osteoblasts, fibroblasts, or dental stem cells and growth factors to achieve the desired goal of enamel, dentin, and periodontal tissue regeneration [134].
- Development of new biofunctionalized CPCs (by incorporating biofunctional agents such as RGD (Arginine–Glycine–Aspartic), Fn (Biofunctional Peptide), FEPP (fibronectin-like engineered polymer protein), Geltrex, and platelets) have shown marked improvements in human umbilical cord-derived mesenchymal stem cells (hUCMSC) proliferation, actin stress fiber density, and osteogenic differentiation. Studies have shown that use of these biofunctionalized BCs shows marked elevation in alkaline phosphatase (ALA), Runx2, Osteocalcin (OC), and collagen I gene expressions and a threefold increase in synthesis of bone mineral matrix with similar mechanical properties as that of cancellous bone. Thus, these stem cell-seeded biofunctionalized BCs are promising to promote bone regeneration in a wide range of dental and craniofacial applications[135].

Collaboration from varied disciplines including basic ceramic research, biochemical research, clinical research, etc., would be required for further improvisation of BCs and making it more functional for its future dental applications [131].

1.12 Conclusion

The development of bioceramics and manufacturing techniques has evolved to become an integral part of the dental health care system. Variations in composition, microstructure, and molecular surface chemistry have broadened the diversity of its application in dentistry. Research is in progress for coupling these materials with tissue engineering ensuring a very bright future for bioceramics in dentistry.

References

1 Bergmann, C.P. and Stumpf, A. (2013). Biomaterials. In: *Dental Ceramics. Topics in Mining, Metallurgy and Materials Engineering*. Berlin, Heidelberg: Springer https://doi.org/10.1007/978-3-642-38224-6_2.

2 Camilleri, J. (2021). Current classification of bioceramic materials in endodontics. In: *Bioceramic Materials in Clinical Endodontics*, 1–6. Switzerland: Springer Nature https://doi.org/10.1007/978-3-030-58170-1_1.

3 Jayaswal, G.P., Dange, S.P., and Khalikar, A.N. (2010). Bioceramic in dental implants: a review. *The Journal of Indian Prosthodontic Society* 10 (1): 8–12. https://doi.org/10.1007/s13191-010-0002-4. Epub 2010 Aug 5. PMID: 23204715; PMCID: PMC3453171.

4 Barbosa, A.V.H., Cazal, C., Nascimento, A.C.A. et al. (2007). Propriedades do cimento Portland e suautilizaçãonaOdontologia: revisão de literatura. *Pesquisa Brasileira em Odontopediatria e Clínica Integrada* 7 (1): 89–94.

5 Peltier, L.F. (1961). The use of plaster of Paris to fill defects in bone. *Clinical Orthopaedics* 21: 1–31. PMID: 14485018.

6 Albee, F.H. (1920). Studies in bone growth: triple calcium phosphate as a stimulus to osteogenesis. *Annals of Surgery* 71 (1): 32–39. https://doi.org/10.1097/00000658-192001000-00006. PMID: 17864220; PMCID: PMC1410453.

7 Ray, R.D. and Ward, A.A. Jr. (1951). A preliminary report on studies of basic calcium phosphate in bone replacement. *Surgical Forum* 429–434.

8 Peltier, L.F. (1959). The use of plaster of Paris to fill large defects in bone. *American Journal of Surgery* 97 (3): 311–315. https://doi.org/10.1016/0002-9610(59)90305-8.

9 Hench, L.L. (1998). Bioceramics. *Journal of the American Ceramic Society* 81 (7): 1705–1728.

10 LeGeros, R., Chohayeb, A., and Shulman, A. (1982). Apatitic calcium phosphates: possible dental restorative materials. *Journal of Dental Research* 61: article 343.

11 Krell, K.F. and Wefel, J.S. (1984). A calcium phosphate cement root canal sealer—scanning electron microscopic analysis. *Journal of Endodontia* 10 (12): 571–576. https://doi.org/10.1016/s0099-2399(84)80103-x.

12 Brown, C. (1987). A new calcium phosphate, water-setting cement. In: *Cements Research Progress 1986* (ed. P.W. Brown), 352–379. Westerville, OH: American Ceramic Society.

13 Lee, S.J., Monsef, M., and Torabinejad, M. (1993). Sealing ability of mineral trioxide aggregate for repair of lateral root perforations. *Journal of Endodontia* 19 (11): 541–544. https://doi.org/10.1016/S0099-2399(06)81282-3.

14 Schmitt, D., Lee, J., and Bogen, G. (2001). Multifaceted use of ProRoot MTA root canal repair material. *Pediatric Dentistry* 23 (4): 326–330. PMID: 11572491.

15 Rahaman, M. (2011). Bioactive glass in tissue engineering. *Acta Biomaterialia* 7 (6): 2355–2373. https://doi.org/10.1016/j.actbio.2011.03.016.

16 Utneja, S., Nawal, R.R., Talwar, S., and Verma, M. (2015). Current perspectives of bio-ceramic technology in endodontics: calcium enriched mixture cement-review of its composition, properties and applications. *Restorative Dentistry and Endodontics* 40: 1–13. https://doi.org/10.5395/rde.2015.40.1.1.

17 Nelea, V., Ristoscu, C., Chiritescu, C. et al. (2000). Pulsed laser deposition of hydroxyapatite thin films on Ti-5Al- 2.5Fe substrates with and without buffer layers. *Applied Surface Science* 168: 127–131. https://doi.org/10.1016/S0169-4332(00)00616-4.

18 Socol G, Torricelli P, lIiescu M, Miroiu F, Bigi A, Werckmann J et al. Biocompatible nanocrystalline octacalcium phosphate thin films obtained by pulsed laser deposition. Biomaterials 2004;25(13):2539–2545. https://doi.org/10.1016/j.biomaterials.2003.09.044

19 Kokubo, T., Ito, S., Sakka, S., and Yamamuro, T. (1986). Formation of a high-strength bioactive glass-ceramic in the system MgO-CaO-SiO2-P2O5. *Journal of Materials Science* 21 (2): 536–540. https://doi.org/10.1007/BF01145520.

20 Floroian, L. (2010). Biocompatibility and physical properties of doped bioactive glass ceramics. *Bulletin of the Transilvania University of Brasov* 3 (52): 27–32.

21 Hench, L.L. and Andersoon, O. (1993). Bioactive glass coatings. In: *An Introduction to Bioceramics* (ed. L.L. Hench and J. Wilson), 239–260. New Jersey: World Scientific Publishing.

22 Sousa, S.R. and Barbosa, M.A. (1996). Effect of hydroxyapatite thickness on metal ion release from Ti6Al4V substrates. *Biomaterials* 17 (4): 397–404. https://doi.org/10.1016/0142-9612(96)89655-4. PMID: 8938233.

23 Santos, J.D., Silva, L.P., Knowles, J.C. et al. (1996). Reinforcement of hydroxyapatite by adding P2O5-CaO glasses with Na2O, K2O and MgO. *Journal of Materials Science. Materials in Medicine* 7: 187–189.

24 Vallet-Regí, M. (2010). Evolution of bioceramics within the field of biomaterials. *Comptes Rendus Chimie* 13 (1–2): 174–185.

25 Best, S.M., Porter, A.E., Thian, E.S., and Huang, J. (2008). Bioceramics: past, present and for the future. *Journal of the European Ceramic Society* 28 (7): 1319–1327. https://doi.org/10.1016/j.jeurceramsoc.2007.12.001.

26 Hench, L.L. and Wilson, J. (1993). *An Introduction to Bioceramics*. Singapore: World Scientific Publ. Co.

27 Hench, L.L. (1991). Bioceramics: from concept to clinic. *Journal of the American Ceramic Society* 74 (7): 1487–1510. https://doi.org/10.1111/j.1151-2916.1991.tb07132.

28 Camilleri, J. (2020). Classification of hydraulic cements used in dentistry. *Frontiers in Dental Medicine* 1: 9. https://doi.org/10.3389/fdmed.2020.00009.

29 Piconi, C. and Porporati, A.A. (2016). Bioinert ceramics: zirconia and alumina. In: *Handbook of Bioceramics and Biocomposites* (ed. I. Antoniac). Cham: Springer https://doi.org/10.1007/978-3-319-12460-5_4.

30 Standard, O. (1995). Application of transformation-toughened zirconia ceramics as bioceramics. PhD thesis, University of New South Wales, Australia.

31 Kay, J.F. (1992). Calcium phosphate coatings for dental implants: current status and future potential. *Dental Clinics of North America* 36 (1): 1–18. https://doi.org/10.1016/S0011-8532(22)02451-X.

32 Torabinejad, M., Hong, C.U., McDonald, F., and Pitt Ford, T.R. (1995). Physical and chemical properties of a new root-end filling material. *Journal of Endodontia* 21 (7): 349–353. https://doi.org/10.1016/S0099-2399(06)80967-2. PMID: 7499973.

33 Kurun Aksoy, M., Tulga Oz, F., and Orhan, K. (2017). Evaluation of calcium (Ca2+) and hydroxide (OH-) ion diffusion rates of indirect pulp capping materials. *The International Journal of Artificial Organs* 40 (11): 641–646. https://doi.org/10.5301/ijao.5000619. Epub 2017 Jul 8. PMID: 28708217.

34 Arias-Moliz, M.T., Farrugia, C., Lung, C.Y.K. et al. (2017). Antimicrobial and biological activity of leachate from light curable pulp capping materials. *Journal of Dentistry* 64: 45–51. https://doi.org/10.1016/j.jdent.2017.06.006. Epub 2017 Jun 20. PMID: 28645637.

35 Camilleri, J., Sorrentino, F., and Damidot, D. (2013). Investigation of the hydration and bioactivity of radiopacified tricalcium silicate cement, biodentine and MTA angelus. *Dental Materials* 29 (5): 580–593. https://doi.org/10.1016/j.dental.2013.03.007. Epub 2013 Mar 26. PMID: 23537569.

36 Raghavendra, S.S., Jadhav, G.R., Gathani, K.M., and Kotadia, P. (2017). Bioceramics in endodontics – a review. *Journal of Istanbul University Faculty of Dentistry* 51 (3 Suppl 1): S128–S137.

37 Shahi, S., Ghasemi, N., Rahimi, S. et al. (2015). The effect of different mixing methods on the pH and solubility of mineral trioxide aggregate and calcium-enriched mixture. *Iranian Endodontic Journal* 10 (2): 140–143.

38 Wang, Z. (2015). Bioceramic materials in endodontics. *Endodontic Topics* 32 (1): 4–30.

39 De Souza, E.T., Nunes Tameirão, M.D., Roter, J.M. et al. (2013). Tridimensional quantitative porosity characterization of three set calcium silicate-based repair cements for endodontic use. *Microscopy Research and Technique* 76 (10): 1093–1098.

40 Kaur, M., Singh, H., Dhillon, J.S. et al. (2017). MTA versus biodentine: review of literature with a comparative analysis. *Journal of Clinical and Diagnostic Research* 11 (8): 1–5.

41 Tuna, E.B., Dinçol, M.E., Gençay, K., and Aktören, O. (2011). Fracture resistance of immature teeth filled with bio aggregate, mineral trioxide aggregate and calcium hydroxide. *Dental Traumatology* 27 (3): 174–178.

42 Saghiri, M.A., Garcia-Godoy, F., Asatourian, A. et al. (2013). Effect of pH on compressive strength of some modification of mineral trioxide aggregate. *Medicina Oral, Patologia Oral y Cirugia Bucal* 18 (4): 714–719.

43 Hashem, A.A. and Amin, S.A. (2012). The effect of acidity on dislodgment resistance of mineral trioxide aggregate and bioaggregate in furcation perforations: an *in vitro* comparative study. *Journal of Endodontia* 38 (2): 245–249.

44 El Sayed, M.A. and Saeed, M.H. (2012). *In vitro* comparative study of sealing ability of Diadent bioaggregate and other root-end filling materials. *Journal of Conservative Dentistry* 15 (3): 249–252.

45 Porter, M.L., Bertó, A., Primus, C.M., and Watanabe, I. (2010). Physical and chemical properties of new-generation endodontic materials. *Journal of Endodontia* 36 (3): 524–528.

46 Parirokh, M. and Torabinejad, M. (2014). Calcium silicate–based cements. In: *Mineral Trioxide Aggregate: Properties and Clinical Applications*, 281–332. Hoboken: Wiley https://doi.org/10.1002/9781118892435.ch10.

47 Hansen, S.W., Marshall, J.G., and Sedgley, C.M. (2011). Comparison of intracanal ERRM and ProRoot MTA to induce pH changes in simulated root resorption defects over 4 weeks in matched pairs of human teeth. *Journal of Endodontia* 37 (4): 502–506.

48 Hirschberg, C.S., Patel, N.S., Patel, L.M. et al. (2013). Comparison of sealing ability of MTA and EndoSequence Bioceramic Root Repair Material: a bacterial leakage study. *Quintessence International* 44 (5): 157–162.

49 Lovato, K.F. and Sedgley, C.M. (2011). Antibacterial activity of EndoSequence root repair material and Proroot MTA against clinical isolates of *Enterococcus faecalis*. *Journal of Endodontia* 37 (11): 1542–1546.

50 Pawan, k., Dehiya, B.S., and Sindhu, A. (2018). Bioceramics for hard tissue engineering applications: a review. *International Journal of Applied Engineering Research* 13 (5): 2744–2752.

51 Thamaraiselvi, T.V. and Rajeswari, S. (2004). Biological evaluation of bioceramic materials – a review. *Biomaterials and Artificial Organs* 18 (1).

52 Sterner, T., Schutze, N., Saxler, G. et al. (2004). Effects of clinically relevant alumina ceramic, zirconia ceramic and titanium particles of different sizes and concentrations on TNF-alpha release in a human macrophage cell line. *Biomedizinische Technik. Biomedical Engineering* 49: 340–344.

53 Josset, Y., Oum'Hamed, Z., Zarrinpour, A. et al. (1999). In vitro reactions of human osteoblasts in culture with zirconia and alumina ceramics. *Journal of Biomedical Materials Research* 47: 481–493.

54 Torricelli, P., Verne´, E., Brovarone, C.V. et al. (2001). Biological glass coating on ceramic materials: in vitro evaluation using primary osteoblast cultures from healthy and osteopenic rat bone. *Biomaterials* 22: 2535–2543.

55 Koh, E.T., McDonald, F., Pitt Ford, T.R., and Torabinejad, M. (1998). Cellular response to mineral trioxide aggregate. *Journal of Endodontia* 24: 543–547.

56 Torabinejad, M., Hong, C.U., Pitt Ford, T.R., and Kettering, J.D. (1995). Cytotoxicity of four root-end filling materials. *Journal of Endodontia* 21: 489–492.

57 Haglund, R., He, J., Jarvis, J. et al. (2003). Effects of root-end filling materials on fibroblasts and macrophages in vitro. *Oral Surgery, Oral Medicine, Oral Pathology, Oral Radiology, and Endodontics* 95: 739–745.

58 Camilleri, J., Montesin, F.E., Di Silvio, L., and Pitt Ford, T.R. (2005). The chemical constitution and biocompatibility of accelerated Portland cement for endodontic use. *International Endodontic Journal* 38: 834–842.

59 Huang, T.H., Ding, S.J., Hsu, T.C., and Kao, C.T. (2003). Effects of mineral trioxide aggregate (MTA) extracts on mitogen-activated protein kinase activity in human osteosarcoma cell line (U2OS). *Biomaterials* 24: 3909–3913.

60 Keiser, K., Johnson, C.C., and Tipton, D.A. (2000). Cytotoxicity of mineral trioxide aggregate using human periodontal ligament fibroblasts. *Journal of Endodontia* 26: 288–291.

61 Camilleri, J. and Pittford, T.R. (2006). Mineral trioxide aggregate: a review of the constituents and biological properties of the material. *IEJ* 39: 747–754.

62 Al, P., Spears, R., Gutmann, J.L., and Opperman, L.A. (2003). Osteoblasts and MG63 osteosarcoma cells behave differently when in contact with ProRootTM MTA and white MTA. *International Endodontic Journal* 36: 564–570.

63 Camilleri, J., Montesin, F.E., Papaioannou, S. et al. (2004). Biocompatibility of two commercial forms of mineral trioxide aggregate. *International Endodontic Journal* 37: 699–704.

64 Abdullah, D., Pitt Ford, T.R., Papaioannou, S. et al. (2002). An evaluation of accelerated Portland cement as a restorative material. *Biomaterials* 23: 4001–4010.

65 Malkondu, Ö., KazandaL, M.K., and Kazazoglu, E. (2014). A review on biodentine, a contemporary dentine replacement and repair material. *BioMed Research International* 2014: Article ID 160951, 10pp. http://dx.doi. org/10.1155/2014/16095.

66 P. Laurent, J. Camps, M. DeM´eo, J. D´ejou, and I. About, "Induction of specific cell responses to a Ca3SiO5-based posterior restorative material," *Dental Materials*, vol. 24, no. 11, pp. 1486–94, 2008.

67 Attik, G.N., Villat, C., Hallay, F. et al. (2014). In vitro biocompatibility of a dentine substitute cement on human MG63 osteoblasts cells: BiodentineTM versus MTA(1). *International Endodontic Journal* 47 (12): 1133–1141.

68 Zhou, H.-M., Shen, Y., Wang, Z.-J. et al. (2013). In vitro cytotoxicity evaluation of a novel root repair material. *Journal of Endodontia* 39 (4): 478–483.

69 Lobo, S.E., Glickman, R., da Silva, W.N. et al. (2015). Response of stem cells from different origins to biphasic calcium phosphate bioceramics. *Cell and Tissue Research* 361 (2): 477–495. https://doi.org/10.1007/s00441-015-2116-9. Epub 2015 Feb 13. PMID: 25676006; PMCID: PMC4529461.

70 Styles, J.A. and Wilson, J. (1976). Comparison between in vitro toxicity of two novel fibrous mineral dusts and their tissue reaction in vivo. *The Annals of Occupational Hygiene* 19: 63–68.

71 Moretton, T.R., Brown, C.E., Legan, J.J., and Kafrawy, A.H. (2000). Tissue reactions after subcutaneous and intraosseous implantation of mineral trioxide aggregate and ethoxybenzoic acid cement. *Journal of Biomedical Materials Research* 52: 528–533.

72 Yaltirik, M., Ozbas, H., Bilgic, B., and Issever, H. (2004). Reactions of connective tissue to mineral trioxide aggregate and amalgam. *Journal of Endodontia* 30: 95–99.

73 Sousa, C.J., Loyola, A.M., Versiani, M.A. et al. (2004). A comparative histological evaluation of the biocompatibility of materials used in apical surgery. *International Endodontic Journal* 37: 738–748.

74 Masuda, Y.M., Wang, X., Hossain, M. et al. (2005). Evaluation of biocompatibility of mineral trioxide aggregate with an improved rabbit ear chamber. *Journal of Oral Rehabilitation* 32: 145–150.

75 Saidon, J., He, J., Zhu, Q. et al. (2003). Cell and tissue reactions to mineral trioxide aggregate and Portland cement. *Oral Surgery, Oral Medicine, Oral Pathology, Oral Radiology, and Endodontics* 95: 483–489.

76 Torabinejad, M., Hong, C.U., Lee, S.J. et al. (1995). Investigation of mineral trioxide aggregate for root end filling in dogs. *Journal of Endodontia* 21: 603–608.

77 Torabinejad, M., Pitt Ford, T.R., McKendry, D.J. et al. (1997). Histologic assessment of Mineral Trioxide Aggregate as root end filling material in monkeys. *Journal of Endodontia* 23: 225–228.

78 Shabahang, S., Torabinejad, M., Boyne, P.P. et al. (1999). A comparative study of root-end induction using osteogenic protein-1, calcium hydroxide, and mineral trioxide aggregate in dogs. *Journal of Endodontia* 25: 1–5.

79 Regan, J.D., Gutmann, J.L., and Witherspoon, D.E. (2002). Comparison of Diaket and MTA when used as root-end filling materials to support regeneration of the periradicular tissues. *International Endodontic Journal* 35: 840–847.

80 Economides, N., Pantelidou, O., Kokkas, A., and Tziafas, D. (2003). Short-term periradicular tissue response to mineral trioxide aggregate (MTA) as root-end filling material. *International Endodontic Journal* 36: 44–48.

81 Apaydin, E.S., Shabahang, S., and Torabinejad, M. (2004). Hard-tissue healing after application of fresh or set MTA as root-endfilling material. *Journal of Endodontia* 30: 21–24.

82 Baek, S.H., Plenk, H., and Kim, S. (2005). Periapical tissue responses and cementum regeneration with amalgam, Super EBA, andMTA as root-end filling materials. *Journal of Endodontia* 31: 444–449.

83 Daculsi, G., LeGeros, R.Z., Nery, E. et al. (1989). Transformation of biphasic calcium phosphate ceramics in vivo: ultrastructural and physicochemical characterization. *Journal of Biomedical Materials Research* 23: 883–894.

84 Ben-Nissan, B. (2014). *Advances in Calcium Phosphate Biomaterials*. Berlin, Germany: Springer.

85 Pitt Ford, T.R., Torabinejad, M., Abedi, H.R. et al. (1996). Using mineral trioxide aggregate as a pulp-capping material. *Journal of the American Dental Association* 127: 1491–1494.

86 Andelin, W.E., Shabahang, S., Wright, K., and Torabinejad, M. (2003). Identification of hard tissue after experimental pulp capping using dentin sialoprotein (DSP) as a marker. *Journal of Endodontia* 29: 646–650.

87 Holland, R., de Souza, V., Murata, S.S. et al. (2001b). Healing process of dog dental pulp after pulpotomy and pulp covering with mineral trioxide aggregate and Portland cement. *Brazilian Dental Journal* 12: 109–113.

88 Menezes, R., Bramante, C.M., Letra, A. et al. (2004). Histologic evaluation of pulpotomies in dog using two types of mineral trioxide aggregate and regular and white Portland cements as wound dressings. *Oral Surgery, Oral Medicine, Oral Pathology, Oral Radiology, and Endodontics* 98: 376–379.

89 Laurent, P., Camps, J., and About, I. (2012). Biodentine(TM) induces TGF-b1 release from human pulp cells and early dental pulp mineraliza- tion. *International Endodontic Journal* 45 (5): 439–448.

90 Zanini, M., Sautier, J.M., Berdal, A., and Simon, S. (2012). Biodentine induces immortalized murine pulp cell differentiation into odontoblast-like cells and stimulates biomineralization. *Journal of Endodontia* 38: 1220–1226.

91 Goldberg, M., Pradelle-Plasse, N., Tran, X.V. et al. (2009). Emerging trends in (bio)material research. In: *Biocompatibility or Cytotoxic Effects of Dental Composites*, 1e.e (ed. M. Goldberg), 181–203. Oxford, UK: Coxmoor Publishing Company.

92 Tran, X.V., Gorin, C., Willig, C. et al. (2012). Effect of a calcium-silicate based restorative cement on pulp repair. *Journal of Dental Research* 91: 1166–1171.

93 Tziafa, C., Koliniotou-Koumpia, E., Papadimitriou, S., and Tziafas, D. (2014). Dentinogenic responses after direct pulp capping of miniature swine teeth with Biodentine. *Journal of Endodontia* 40 (12): 1967–1971.

94 Mathieu, S., Jeanneau, C., Sheibat-Othman, N. et al. (2013). Usefulness of controlled release of growth factors in investigating the early events of dentin-pulp regeneration. *Journal of Endodontia* 39 (2): 228–235.

95 Shayegan, A., Jurysta, C., Atash, R. et al. (2012). Biodentine used as a pulp-capping agent in primary pig teeth. *Pediatric Dentistry* 34 (7): e202–e208.

96 Luo, Z., Li, D., Kohli, M.R. et al. (2014). Effect of Biodentine on the proliferation, migration and adhesion of human dental pulp stem cells. *Journal of Dentistry* 42 (4): 490–497.

97 Boyde, A. and Jones, S.J. (1983). Backscattered electronimaging of dental tissues. *Anatomy and Embryology* 168: 211–226.

98 LeGeros, R.Z., Orly, I., LeGeros, J.P. et al. (1988). Scanning electron microscopy and electron probe microanalyses of the crystalline components of human and animal dental calculi. *Scanning Microscopy* 2: 345–356.

99 Jean, A.H., Pouezat, J.A., and Daculsi, G. (1993). Pulpal response to calcium phosphate materials. In vivo study of calcium phosphate materials in endodontics. *Cells & Materials* 3 (2): Article 7.

100 Rimondini, L., Cerroni, L., Carrassi, A., and Torricelli, P. (2002). Bacterial colonization of zirconia ceramic surfaces: An *in vitro* and *in vivo* study. *The International Journal of Oral & Maxillofacial Implants* 17: 793–798.

101 Al-Hezaimi, K., Al-Shalan, T.A., Naghshbandi, J. et al. (2006). Antibacterial effect of two mineral trioxide aggregate (MTA) preparations against *Enterococcus faecalis* and *Streptococcus sanguis in vitro. Journal of Endodontia* 32: 1053–1056.

102 Torabinejad, M., Hong, C.U., Pitt Ford, T.R., and Kettering, J.D. (1995). Antibacterial effects of some root end filling materials. *Journal of Endodontia* 21: 403–406.

103 Bhavana, V., Chaitanya, K.P., Gandi, P. et al. (2015). Evaluation of antibacterial and antifungal activity of new calcium-based cement (Biodentine) compared to MTA and glass ionomer cement. *Journal of Conservative Dentistry* 18: 44–46.

104 Asgary, S., Akbari Kamrani, F., and Taheri, S. (2007). Evaluation of antimicrobial effect of MTA, calcium hydroxide, and CEM cement. *Iranian Endodontic Journal* 2: 105–109.

105 Koruyucu, M., Topcuoglu, N., Tuna, E.B. et al. (2015). An assessment of antibacterial activity of three pulp capping materials on *Enterococcus faecalis* by a direct contact test: an *in vitro* study. *European Journal of Dentistry* 9: 240–245.

106 Esteki, P., Jahromi, M.Z., and Tahmourespour, A. (2021). *In vitro* antimicrobial activity of mineral trioxide aggregate, Biodentine and calcium-enriched mixture cement against *Enterococcus faecalis*, *Streptococcus mutans* and *Candida albicans* using the agar diffusion technique. *Dental Research Journal* 18: 3.

107 Khan, A.S. and Syed, M.R. (2019). A review of BCs-based dental restorative materials. *Dental Materials Journal* 38 (2): 163–176.

108 Gupta, A.D. (2020). Endodontic treatment of immature tooth – a challenge. *Journal of Pre-Clinical and Clinical Research* 14 (3): 73–79.

109 Wang, W., Liao, S., Zhu, Y. et al. (2015). Recent applications of nanomaterials in prosthodontics. *Journal of Nanomaterials* 1: 1–11.

110 Leal, F., De-Deus, G., Brandão, C. et al. (2011). Comparison of the root-end seal provided by BC repair cements and white MTA. *International Endodontic Journal* 44 (7): 662–668.

111 Moreira Filho, O., Wykrota, F.H., and Lobo, S.E. (2021). Restoring facial contour and harmony using biphasic calcium phosphate bioceramics. *PRSGO* 9 (4): e3516.

112 Ramadoss, R., Padmanaban, R., and Subramanian, B. (2022). Role of bioglass in enamel remineralization: existing strategies and future prospects—a narrative review. *Journal of Biomedical Materials Research Part B: Applied Biomaterials Journal* 110 (1): 45–66.

113 Abbassy, M.A., Bakry, A.S., and Hill, R. (2021). The efficiency of fluoride bioactive glasses in protecting enamel surrounding orthodontic bracket. *BioMed Research International* 25 (3): 5544196.

114 Nery, E.B., Lynch, K.L., Hirthe, W.M., and Mueller, K.H. (1975). BC implants in surgically produced infrabony defects. *Journal of Periodontology* 46 (6): 328–347.

115 Wu, Y., Woodbine, L., Carr, A.M. et al. (2020). 3D printed calcium phosphate cement (CPC) scaffolds for anti-cancer drug delivery. *Pharmaceutics* 12 (11): 1077.

116 Arcos, D. and Vallet-Regi, M. (2013). Bioceramics for drug delivery. *Acta Materialia* 61 (3): 890–911.

117 Yu, X., Tang, X., Gohil, S.V., and Laurencin, C.T. (2015). Biomaterials for bone regenerative engineering. *Advanced Healthcare Materials* 4 (9): 1268–1285.

118 Lee, T.M., Chang, E., Wang, B.C., and Yang, C.Y. (1996 Feb). Characteristics of plasma-sprayed bioactive glass coatings on Ti-6A1-4V alloy: an in vitro study. *Surface and Coatings Technology SURF* 79 (1-3): 170–177.

119 Prati, C. and Gandolfi, M.G. (2015). Calcium silicate bioactive cements: biological perspectives and clinical applications. *Dental Materials Journal* 31 (4): 351–370.

120 Jain, P. and Ranjan, M. (2015). The rise of biocramics in endodontics: a review. *International Journal of Pharma and Bio Sciences* 6 (1): 416–422.

121 Salmasi, S., Nayyer, L., Seifalian, A.M., and Blunn, G.W. (2016). M8: nanohydroxyapatite effect on the degradation, osteoconduction and mechanical properties of polymeric bone tissue engineered scaffolds. *Open Journal of Orthopedics* 10: 900–909.

122 Wang, W. and Yeung, K.W. (2017). Bone grafts and biomaterials substitutes for bone defect repair: a review. *Bioactive Materials* 2 (4): 224–247.

123 Wang, S.H., Shih, W.J., Li, W.L. et al. (2005). Morphology of calcium phosphate coatings deposited on a Ti–6Al–4V substrate by an electrolytic method under 80 Torr. *Journal of the European Ceramic Society* 25 (14): 3287–3292.

124 Shao, H., Sun, M., Zhang, F. et al. (2018). Custom repair of mandibular bone defects with 3D printed BC scaffolds. *Journal of Dental Research* 97 (1): 68–76.

125 Koch, K. and Brave, D. (2009). The increased use of BCs in endodontics. *Dentaltown* 10 (4): 39–43.

126 Chitra, S. and Balakumar, S. (2021). Insight into the impingement of different sodium precursors on structural, biocompatible, and hemostatic properties of bioactive materials. *Materials Science and Engineering* 123 (4): 111959.

127 Bargavi, P., Ramya, R., Chitra, S. et al. (2020). Bioactive, degradable and multi-functional three-dimensional membranous scaffolds of bioglass and alginate composites for tissue regenerative applications. *Biomaterials Science* 8 (4): 4003–4025.

128 Kasuga, T. (2005). Bioactive calcium pyrophosphate glasses and glass-ceramics. *Acta Biomaterialia* 1 (1): 55–64.

129 Zapf, A.M., Chedella, S.C., and Berzins, D.W. (2015). Effect of additives on mineral trioxide aggregate setting reaction product formation. *Journal of Endodontia* 41 (1): 88–91.

130 Ishikawa, K., Mazuyi, S., Miyamoto, Y., and Kawate, K. (2003). Bioengeenering. In: *Comprehensive Structural Integrity*, vol. 1 (ed. I. Milne, B. Karihaloo, and R.O. Richie), 169–214. Elsevier.

131 Kawahara, H. (1987). BCs for hard tissue replacements. *Clinical Materials* 2 (3): 181–206.

132 Truong, L.B., Medina Cruz, D., Mostafavi, E. et al. (2021). Advances in 3D-printed surface-modified Ca-Si BC structures and their potential for bone tumor therapy. *Materials* 14 (14): 3844.

133 Tan B, Tang Q, Zhong Y, Wei Y, He L, Wu Y etal. Biomaterial-based strategies for maxillofacial tumour therapy and bone defect regeneration. International Journal of Oral Science 2021;13(1):1–6.

134 Sowmya, S., Bumgardener, J.D., Chennazhi, K.P. et al. (2013). Role of nanostructured biopolymers and bioceramics in enamel, dentin and periodontal tissue regeneration. *Progress in Polymer Science* 38 (10): 1748–1772.

135 Thein-Han, W., Liu, J., and Xu, H.H. (2012). Calcium phosphate cement with biofunctional agents and stem cell seeding for dental and craniofacial bone repair. *Dental Materials* 28 (10): 1059–1070.

2

Calcium Silicate-Based Dental Bioceramics: History, Status, and Future

Abubaker Qutieshat, Shahab Javanmardi, and Gurdeep Singh

Adult Restorative Dentistry, Oman Dental College, Muscat, Oman

CONTENTS

Bioceramics in Endodontics, First Edition. Edited by Viresh Chopra.
© 2024 John Wiley & Sons, Inc. Published 2024 by John Wiley & Sons, Inc.
Companion website: www.wiley.com/go/chopra/bioceramicsinendodontics

2.1 Introduction

Dental bioceramics based on calcium silicate are a type of material that belong to the category of regenerative bioactive materials. Conventional type 1 Portland cement served as the foundation for the very first commercially available calcium silicate-based dental bioceramic. Their superior sealing ability, regenerative capabilities, and antibacterial properties have led to an increase in their application in contemporary endodontic procedures. However, because of factors such as cost, handling properties, extended setting time (during which they run the risk of being washed out of their placement site), concerns over potentially harmful elements contained in the material, and aesthetic considerations, researchers nowadays are developing calcium silicate-based materials that are more user-friendly. Enhancing calcium silicate-based materials has involved the removal of potentially toxic elements, the engineering of the materials' particle size, the addition of setting accelerants, mixing and flow enhancing polymers, and stabilization mixing gels. All these methods have been effectively utilized in the creation of some newer formulations which are demonstrating a tremendous amount of potential in terms of replacing the conventional types that are currently on the market.

The chemical elements used to make calcium silicate-based bioceramic materials are only a small subset of the periodic table, consisting of silicon, a metalloid, and calcium, an alkaline earth metal. After a specific need has been identified, the process of developing a new calcium silicate-based material begins. Following that, an idea for a potential material is developed with the goal of using the new material in dental applications. It is only after selecting the appropriate chemical composition in conjunction with structural and compositional controls that it is determined whether the new biomaterial is suitable or not, and this only after a lengthy cycle of trial and error. A common occurrence in materials science nowadays is that when an improvement in certain chemical and biological properties is achieved from one perspective, it may result in a negative effect on the physical parameters of the material in question from another perspective, which poses a significant challenge. In this chapter, we aim to provide an up-to-date view of calcium silicate-based materials and to provide the reader with the opportunity to acquire a better understanding of the temporal changes that occur in material properties whenever a compositional change is implemented.

The current reliance on the capacity of cells to tolerate cytotoxic substances will be replaced as the new standard of measurement with the capacity of tissues to regenerate themselves. Therefore, the utilization of bioactive materials in dental work will become more prevalent in the future.

2.2 Bioceramics: The What and the Why

Ceramics are produced when compounds, either metallic or nonmetallic, are subjected to high temperatures to facilitate their combination into a single substance [1]. This ultimately results in the formation of a material complex that is made up of the individual compounds being sintered together into a single entity. Bioceramics are any ceramics that are used in the treatment, reconstruction, or repair of diseased or damaged components of the musculoskeletal system. The term "bioceramics" refers to any ceramics that fall under this category. In addition, they can be bioinert (like zirconia), bioresorbable (like tricalcium phosphate), bioactive (like hydroxyapatite), bioconductive (like porous hydroxyapatite coated ceramics), or any combination of these properties [2].

2.3 Endodontic Repair Materials with Ideal Properties

Periodontal tissue is frequently brought into direct and consistent contact with various endodontic materials. The perfect material would be dimensionally stable, nontoxic, and free of carcinogens. It would also prevent the leakage of microorganisms and the associated microbial by-products; it would be biocompatible with tissue fluid; and it would prevent leakage [3, 4]. Regeneration of tissue complexes, ease of use, and visibility of the material on radiographs are now also included as desirable properties of the material [5].

Throughout the years, numerous materials have been investigated, tried, and evaluated for use as root-end fillings and for repairing perforations in the root canal system. Studies on the biocompatibility, microleakage, and handling characteristics of a variety of materials that have historically been used in perforation and periradicular surgery have shown that there is not one material that is the master of all. Instead, the studies have shown that some materials are adequate for some tasks, but not for all applications. The fact that the tissues in which materials are implanted are able to tolerate those materials is the best that can be said about those materials. Cell viability assays have been used to determine biocompatibility and bioactivity, as have investigations of genotoxicity [6, 7].

2.4 Calcium Silicate-based Materials: A Look Back in History

In the April issue of the Deutsche Vierteljahrsschrift für Zahnheilkunde (German Quarterly for Dentistry) in 1878, a dentist named Witte from Hanover, Germany, reported a new method for filling root canals with Portland cement [8]. He praised the method and said it should be used by all dentists. According to the report, Portland cement is finely ground before being stored in a corked bottle to prepare it for dental applications (Figure 2.1). As per Witte's instructions, and in describing the once novel method back then, a small amount of creosote or carbolic acid and a few drops of water mixed with Portland cement make the cement workable and gradually change its color from ash-gray to dark brown. The mixture is then placed on a serviette to absorb any excess liquid. After the canal that needs to be filled has

Dr. Witte: Das Füllen der Wurzelcanäle mit Portland-Cement. 153

Das Füllen der Wurzelcanäle mit Portland-Cement.

Von

Dr. **Witte** in Hannover.

Ich fülle seit einem halben Jahre Wurzelcanäle mit soge-nanntem Portland- oder Buxtehuder Cement und habe seitdem keine Klagen über Wurzelhautentzündungen gehört. Ich lasse mir einen Theil Portland-Cement recht fein reiben und hebe ihn, in einem Fläschchen wohl verkorkt, zum Gebrauche auf. Sobald ich nun einen Wurzelcanal zu füllen habe, thue ich von diesem Cement ein Wenig auf eine Glasplatte, tupfe etwas Creosot oder Carbolsäure und etwas Wasser auf die Platte und rühre Alles zusammen. Dann lege ich diesen Brei auf eine Serviette und drücke ein Wenig das überflüssige Wasser aus, dann halte ich den zu füllenden Zahn so viel wie möglich trocken, trockne Zahn und Wurzeln aus, stopfe den angemischten Cement in die Wur-zeln hinein und lege etwas Zunder zum Trockenhalten darauf. Nach einigen Minuten nehme ich den Zunder wieder heraus und reinige den Zahn von dem überflüssigen Cement, der mittlerweile schon ziemlich hart geworden ist, trockne alsdann nochmals den Zahn aus und fülle ihn mit Gold u. s. w.

Dieser Cement bindet alle Flüssigkeiten, die in der Zahn-wurzel sind, und bildet mit ihnen in Verbindung mit dem Creosot eine unauflösliche, harte Masse.

Figure 2.1 A snippet from Witte's paper as it appeared in the April issue of the Deutsche Vierteljahrsschrift für Zahnheilkunde (German Quarterly for Dentistry) in 1878 [8].

dried, the cement is placed inside and covered with gauze for a few minutes to dry. Then, the gauze is removed, the excess cement is removed, and the access cavity is sealed with gold restoration. Witte believed that using this cement as a root canal filling produced better results than using any of the other materials available during his time, such as zinc chloride, which easily corroded, gold, which caused problems because it was a heat conductor, or cotton, which would likely rot.

Interestingly, Witte appears to have reported a case of vital pulp therapy in his paper when attempting to treat a very deep cavity close to the pulp, or what is now known as an irreversibly inflamed tooth. He first tried to treat the patient by filling the deep cavity with amalgam, which caused severe pain, and this is when he decided to use his "novel" method (i.e. by using Portland cement), which resulted in a favorable outcome and the absence of any symptoms for an extended period of time [8].

Schlenker reviewed Witte's technique two years later and published a paper titled "Filling the root canals with Portland cement according to Dr. Witte" that proposes some modifications to Witte's original technique [9] (Figure 2.2). It was reported that Witte's mixture is friable, making its application into the root canal difficult. It was also reported that the crumbly mixture could not completely fill the root canal space. The suggested modification is to pour one or two drops of carbolic acid (not creosote) on a clean glass slab and then pour what runs off back into the bottle. After that, one drop of water is added. Following the mixing of these two liquids, cement is added and mixed to a consistency that does not crumble but is also not too flowy. The mixture is then transferred into the root canal

---

Das Füllen der Wurzelkanäle mit Portland-Cement nach Dr. Witte.

Von

M. Schlenker.

Bekanntlich machte uns der College Dr. Witte in Hannover im Aprilhefte 1878 auf seine oben angeführte Operationsmethode aufmerksam, indem er dieselbe als ausgezeichnet schildert und zur Nachahmung empfiehlt. Dr. Witte lässt sich diesen Portland-

xx.   19

Figure 2.2 A snippet from Schlenker's paper as it appeared in the January issue of the Deutsche Vierteljahrsschrift für Zahnheilkunde (German Quarterly for Dentistry) in 1880 [9].

space with a small excavator. As per Schlenker's instructions, and in describing the modified Witte's method, the first addition should be pushed deep into the canal with a tweezer-held small cotton pellet. The cotton pellet can be left inside to absorb excess water before being removed to apply the second and subsequent additions. The excess cement is removed, and the cement filling is capped with zinc phosphate before being thoroughly washed with water to remove any remaining zinc phosphate cement before introducing the gold restoration. Interestingly, Schlenker warned of the risk of tooth discoloration if excess Portland cement is not removed. In this modified technique, zinc phosphate cement is added to provide the required seal that Portland cement would not provide because of its porous nature.

Schlenker reported the use of Portland cement on 25 teeth with a one-year follow-up and a 100% success rate. It is worth noting that in the study, success was defined as the absence of symptoms and/or infection. The Portland cement material tended to stain anterior teeth, which was the only negative outcome reported among the 25 treated cases (Figure 2.3). As a result, it is safe to assume that this was the first non-randomized, non-controlled study ever conducted on a calcium silicate-based material [9].

It is worth noting, however, that carbolic acid and creosote was commonly used in root canal treatment back in the nineteenth century [10]. However, when the first reports of their toxicity began to emerge, these materials were identified as poisonous and their use began to decline significantly [11]. This could be why any further development on Portland cement was halted, because the materials suggested by Witte to serve as a vehicle were prohibited from being used in dental applications, effectively putting Portland cement development on hold until the first reports of development began to emerge in the 1990s at Loma Linda University [12].

Carbolic acid and creosote solutions in concentrations ranging from 1 to 5% were thought to have stimulating and antiseptic effects when applied to an exposed pulp, facilitating the stoppage of inflammation and preventing necrosis of the remaining vital part of the pulp [13].

2.5 Chemical Properties

Mineral trioxide aggregate (MTA) refers to the first experimental calcium silicate-based dental bioceramic developed in modern times [14]. Torabinejad at Loma Linda University introduced a modified Portland cement as an endodontic material and patented it as mineral trioxide aggregate (MTA) in the 1990s. In 1998, it was approved by the US Food and Drug Administration and became commercially available as ProRoot MTA (Figure 2.4). When compared to the one used by

Wurzelfüllungen mit Portland-Cement nach Witte.

Nr.	Name, Alter und Beruf	Constitution	Zahngattung	Zeit der Application der Pasta	Zeit der Extraction der Pulpa	Zeit der Füllung	Füllungs-Material	Bemerkungen
1.	Hr. G., Zeichner, 30 J. alt.	gesund.	u. l. Sap.	9/III.	15/III.	15/III.	Pouls. N. M.-Pl.	Der Zahn wurde vor 2 Jahren von einem Collegen als „nicht füllbar" dem Schicksal überlassen.
2.	desgl.	—	ob. l. 1. Mol.	desgl.	desgl.	desgl.	desgl.	desgl.
3.	L. Müller, 40 J. alt.	robust.	u. r. Cusp.	—	—	12/III.	Gold.	Wurde vor mehreren Jahren nach vorausgegangener Cauterisation mit Amalgam gefüllt, Pulpa aber sitzen gelassen, weshalb bei jed. Witterungswechsel Schmerz (Periostitis) auftrat.
4.	D. O., Dir., 45 J. alt.	robust.	u. r. 1. Bicusp.	12/III.	16/III.	16/III.	Amalgam.	
5.	desgl.	—	u. r. 2. Bicusp.	desgl.	desgl.	desgl.	desgl.	Pulpa reagirte in der Wurzelspitze noch.

Nr.	Name, Alter und Beruf	Constitution	Zahngattung	Zeit der Application der Pasta	Zeit der Extraction der Pulpa	Zeit der Füllung	Füllungs-Material	Bemerkungen
6.	V., Fabrikant, 30 Jahre alt.	gesund.	ob. r. 1. Mol.	—	—	12/III.	Amalgam.	Pulpazersetzt. Pat. suchte infolge periodisch auftretender Periostitis Hilfe.
7.	D. G., Dir., 45 J. alt.	robust.	ob. l. 2. Bicusp.	13/III.	14/III.	16/III.	desgl.	
8.	desgl.	—	ob. r. 2. Bicusp.	desgl.	desgl.	desgl.	desgl.	
9.	Frl. N. M., 40 J. alt.	anämisch.	u. r. 1. Bicusp.	15/III.	16/III.	16/III.	desgl.	
10.	desgl.	—	u. r. 2. Bicusp.	desgl.	desgl.	desgl.	desgl.	
11.	Frl. M., Kelln., 32 J. alt.	zart.	u. r. 1. Mol.	15. u. 16/III.	17/III.	19/III.	desgl.	
12.	desgl.	—	u. l. 1. Bicusp.	15/III.	desgl.	desgl.	desgl.	
13.	T. L., Weinh., 35 J. alt.	gesund.	ob. l. Central-schneidezahn.	—	—	19/III.	Gold.	Pulpa wurde vor 2 Jahren zerstört.
14.	Frl. N., Lehrerin, 27 J. alt.	klein, gesund.	u. l. Cusp.	17/III.	18/III.	25/III.	Pouls. N. M.-Pl.	
15.	Sch., Fabrikant, 30 J. alt.	kräftig.	ob. r. 1. Bicusp.	—	—	17/III.	desgl.	Wurde vor 2 J. von einem Pariser Collegen unter Zurücklassung d. caut. Pulpa m. Hill's Stopping gefüllt. Periostitis.

Nr.	Name, Alter und Beruf	Constitution	Zahngattung	Zeit der Application der Pasta	Zeit der Extraction der Pulpa	Zeit der Füllung	Füllungs-Material	Bemerkungen
16.	Sch., Fabrikant, 30 J. alt.	kräftig.	u. l. 2. Bicusp.	—	—	17/III.	Amalgam.	Der Grund der Cavität war noch bedeckt mit Hill's Stopping; im Kanale eine kleine Baumwollpille. Dieser Zahn hat nie geschmerzt.
17.	F. Milcher, 19 J. alt.	Schwerhörigkeit.	ob. l. 1. Bicusp.	20/III.	21/III.	25/III.	desgl.	
18.	desgl.	—	ob. r. 1. Bicusp.	desgl.	desgl.	desgl.	desgl.	
19.	Frl. St., 40 J. alt.	zart, vorsteh. Oberkiefer.	ob. l. Cusp.	—	20/III.	20/III.	Pouls. N. M.-Pl.	Pulpa abgestorben.
20.	H. Schmid, 39 J. alt.	corpulent, untersetzt.	ob. l. Mol.	21/III.	22/III.	29/III.	desgl.	Eine vorhandene leichte Periostitis heilte in 5 Tagen.
21.	Frl. K., 18 J. alt.	anämisch.	ob. l. Seitenschneidezahn.	—	—	21/III.	desgl.	Pulpa abgestorben.
22.	Frau M., 27 J. alt.	nervös.	ob. l. 1. Bicusp.	25/III.	26/III.	3/IV.	Amalgam.	Sehr zu Abscessbildung geneigt. Vor 2 Jahren musste infolge dessen der 1. Seitenschneidezahn (mit Gold gefüllt) extrahirt werden.
23.	desgl.	—	ob. r. 1. Bicusp.	desgl.	desgl.	desgl.	desgl.	
24.	desgl.	—	ob. r. Cusp.	desgl.	desgl.	desgl.	desgl.	
25.	Jgfr. M. H., 21 J. alt.	gesund.	u. l. 1. Mol.	26/III.	27/III.	30/III.	desgl.	

Figure 2.3 A snippet from Schlenker's non-randomized non-controlled study results conducted in 1880 using Portland cement as a root canal filling material [9].

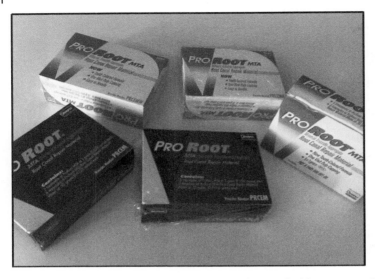

Figure 2.4 The first commercial form of gray mineral trioxide aggregate (brown pack) and white mineral trioxide aggregate (white pack).

Witte in 1878, the original material is essentially a refined version of ordinary gray Portland cement, and it contains an additional component known as bismuth oxide (a metal oxide that gives MTA its radiopacity). Portland cement is primarily derived from calcite, a naturally occurring calcium carbonate that accounts for more than three-quarters of the raw materials mix used in the production of Portland cement clinker. While the primary calcium-rich raw material may contain significant impurities, a secondary raw material is usually required to provide enough bulk. Typically, this secondary material is clay (argil) or shale [15]. Five years after FDA approval, a study compared Portland cement and MTA and found no significant differences in the elemental constituents of either, with the exception of the addition of bismuth oxide [16, 17].

The preferred formula for MTA, according to its US patents, was based on the commercially available "Colton Fast-Set" brand of cement manufactured by the California Portland Cement Company (Torabinejad and White, 1995).

The presence of calcium phosphate was reported in the first research paper on the constituents of MTA (Loma Linda University) in 1995, authored by the new material's creators [12]. However, using energy dispersive analysis with X-ray, Asgary et al. were unable to detect the presence of phosphorus [18]. Camilleri et al. also demonstrated that MTA was devoid of phosphorus [19]. Both of these reports raised concerns among scientists about the accuracy of the 1995 paper. However, subsequent investigations discovered phosphorus levels in MTA products to be very low, near the detection limit of electron probe microanalysis [20, 21], which still did not correlate with the manufacturer's material safety data sheet [22]. Because it is unlikely that there has been a significant compositional change in MTA materials since the first report, and because Portland cement is primarily composed of silicate and aluminate materials [15, 20, 21], earlier reports [12] of MTA phosphorus content are incorrect [18].

It was later found that the MTA samples reported by Torabinjead in his 1995 paper [12] had been contaminated by prior immersion in phosphate solution [23]. Later, confirming Asgary's and Camilleri's research teams' concerns, it was confirmed that the MTA powder is primarily composed of tricalcium and dicalcium silicates, as well as bismuth oxide. Analysis by X-ray diffraction revealed that the cement was completely crystalline, with distinct peaks attributable to distinct phases [19].

As was mentioned earlier, Portland cement is primarily derived from limestone (calcite), with clay and shale serving as secondary raw materials. The raw materials are first crushed, ground, and combined in the desired proportions before being heated in a rotary kiln at temperatures ranging from 1400 to 1600 °C. The high levels of heat cause the limestone and clay/shale to break down into the fundamental raw materials, which can then be combined to produce cement clinker. Calcination is the process of transforming raw materials into clinker for use in the cement manufacturing process. The clinker that is produced as a by-product is allowed to cool, then ground into a powder. After that, gypsum is added to slow down the setting time of the Portland cement that was produced as a result [15]. After calcination, the main constituents of cement clinker are tri- and dicalcium silicate (alite and belite), tetra-calcium aluminoferrite (ferrite), tricalcium aluminate (aluminate or celite), and calcium sulphate dihydrate (gypsum) [24].

MTA in its gray form was responsible for the discoloration of tissues and teeth, which led to the development of the white variant of MTA [25]. As is the case with gray MTA, the elemental components of white MTA do not display any significant differences from those of white Portland cement, with the exception of the presence of bismuth oxide [16]. Despite this, both forms of MTA have been linked to discoloration, which has been attributed to the materials' characteristic slow hydrating process. This process allows for the absorption and subsequent hemolysis of erythrocytes from the adjacent tissues, which ultimately leads to discoloration of the material and the tooth [25, 26]. The percentage of aluminum oxide, magnesium oxide, and in particular ferrous oxide in gray MTA is significantly higher than it is in the white variant. Both gray variants of ordinary Portland cement and MTA take on a gray hue because of the presence of tricalcium aluminoferrite, and these characteristics sum up the primary distinctions between the two varieties of cement [23].

2.5.1 Heavy Metal Contamination

It was found that gray Portland cement had higher levels of heavy metals than white Portland cement and both variants of MTA, with levels of arsenic and lead being of particular concern [27]. Although favorable constituent analysis and bio-compatibility results have been demonstrated using commercial forms of both variants of Portland cement, some authors have even commented that it would be unwise to use commercial Portland cements because of potentially unsafe levels of arsenic [28]. However, in another study, it was found that arsenic levels were comparable between several types of Portland cement and MTA [29]. It was reported that the levels of arsenic in both varieties of MTA were lower than the 2-ppm safety level required by the ISO standard or dental water-based cements [30]. Interestingly, Camilleri found that arsenic concentrations were higher than those allowed by the ISO standard, but that effective release in a simulated tissue fluid was found to be negligible [31]. However, it is important to note that none of the formulations that were reported to contain high levels of arsenic were MTA's pre-cursor, which was the "Colton Fast-Set" brand of cement that was produced by the California Portland Cement Company.

On a separate but related front, concerns about the toxicity of aluminum and its association with autism and Alzheimer's disease have led to the production of calcium silicate cements that do not contain the aluminate phase that is present in MTA-based cements [32]. Biodentine, BioAggregate, EndoSequence, NeoMTA Plus, iRoot BP Plus, and BioRoot RCS are relatively new calcium silicate cements that were manufactured in a laboratory without the presence of an aluminate phase [33]. Biodentine and BioAggregate cements have shown arsenic levels that are comparable to those of Portland cement and MTA [31]. Furthermore, when the acid-soluble trace element content of each was investigated, Biodentine contained a high concentration of lead, whereas BioAggregate contained a high concentration of chromium [34].

Since the introduction of the sol–gel production method, there has been an increase in the quantity of calcium silicates that are chemically pure. This approach enables the synthesis of cements that have a higher purity at lower processing temperatures, as well as improved control over the structural homogeneity of the final product. For instance, the MTA-based materials no longer require the utilization of raw materials such as limestone and clay as part of their development. This manufacturing process has the potential to be completely implemented in the near future for the purpose of the production of superior calcium silicate cements [35].

The fineness of Portland cement is measured by surface area and is indicated by the Blaine number (measurement of surface area per gram of material) of the cement. A typical Portland cement has a Blaine number in the 320–550 m^2/kg range, with some manufacturers producing finer particle sizes and others producing larger particle sizes [15]. According to the material's US patents, the preferred Blaine number for MTA is between 450 and 460 m^2/kg, indicating that some ordinary Portland cement formulations used in the construction industry have finer particle size than MTA [36]. This also correlates to the fact that the source from which Portland cement-based material is produced is critical in determining its suitability for use in dental applications.

Particle size comparisons of commercial MTA variants reveal differences between color variants and manufacturers. When it comes to color differences, white MTA has smaller particles and a narrower particle size range than gray MTA. In terms of manufacturer differences, ProRoot MTA has coarser particle size overall, but with more circularity and fewer extra-large particles than MTA Angelus. ProRoot MTA also has a very similar particle size distribution compared to ordinary Portland cement [37]. The clinical significance of this is that particle size and shape may affect hydration and mineral release from calcium silicate-based cements.

2.5.2 Setting Reaction

The process of setting calcium silicate-based cements is a dynamic cascade-like process. The rate at which the process of hydration occurs varies depending on the ratios of the elementary components. Experimental work in the field of dentistry has focused mainly on analyzing the end products rather than addressing specific dynamics of the setting reaction, therefore, the dental literature does not contain a description that can be taken as definitive of the setting process. Comparisons to the setting of Portland cement have been used to explain the various phases of hydration; however, specific interactions with phosphate-containing tissue fluids produce specific differences between the setting of Portland cement and calcium silicate-based dental cements via hydration with water alone, and a biological system in the presence of phosphate-containing tissue fluids. When calcium silicate cements are wet, a dynamic hydration reaction takes place, and the various material phases hydrate at different rates at the same time. In the initial reaction, calcium oxide hydrates rapidly forming calcium hydroxide. Tricalcium aluminate hydrates shortly after the hydration of calcium oxide [38].

As a result, the setting reaction of Portland cement-based calcium silicate cements can be simply summed up as the production of a mixed hydrated calcium aluminate, calcium sulphate aluminate, and amorphous hydrated calcium silicate matrix. This matrix is the final product of the setting reaction. The matrix also contains calcium hydroxide in excess, which can be found in crystalline form dispersed throughout the material. The findings of studies using scanning electron microscopy also confirm this complicated mixture of mineral phases. It is possible to observe bismuth oxide randomly dispersed throughout the hydrated matrix when it is utilized as a radioopacifier [39].

The ability of Portland cement-based materials to form calcium hydroxide as a hydration product and hydroxyapatite in the presence of phosphates makes these materials bioactive [40]. Oral physiological fluids contain a high concentration of phosphate ions, which facilitate the hydration reaction that leads to the formation of carbonate calcium phosphate. The same physicochemical reactions can occur when the materials are immersed in culture medium containing a phosphate source [41]. When Portland cement reacts with phosphate ions, an amorphous calcium phosphate phase forms, which eventually hydrolyzes to form an apatite phase [42]. Amorphous calcium phosphate is a well-known intermediate compound that precedes the appearance of biological apatites in skeletal calcification [43]. Because the maximum pH in Portland cement can reach greater than 9 when in contact with physiological fluids, this amorphous transformation occurs by the preferential formation of apatite rather than octacalcium phosphate, as is the case in a phosphate-free medium [42, 44]. Because the hydroxyl ions are incorporated in the hydroxyl sites of the apatites, the continuous pH drop after reaching maximum pH in the Portland cement/physiological fluid reflects this transformation [45]. The specific reaction responsible for this precipitation may be the following, which is a well-known reaction in any biologic calcification process [34, 46]:

$$10Ca^{+2} + 6\left(PO_4\right)^{-3} + 2\left(OH\right)^- \rightarrow Ca_{10}\left(PO_4\right)_6\left(OH\right)_2$$

This reaction occurs in vivo and in vitro with many calcium-containing materials in contact with biologic environments [34]. An essentially similar reaction is also responsible for the formation of the adherent hydroxyapatite layer that appears on the MTA and Portland cement surfaces when in contact with physiological fluids. According to several studies, the material precipitating on the surface of white and gray MTA is hydroxyapatite [20, 47]. As a result, in the presence of phosphate ions, Portland cement is potentially bioactive, which may be attributed to the formation of apatites. Tay et al. were among the first to report apatite precipitation using white Portland cement [42]. A similar formation was observed on the interface between all Portland cement-based materials and dentin because of calcium ion release from the cement reacting with phosphates from the simulated tissue fluid. The resultant apatites are very similar to those biological apatite phases found in bone, cementum, and dentin [46]. Although the Portland cement's in vitro bioactivity may be attributed to its ability to produce biologically compatible apatites, additional experiments are required to determine what actually stimulates cell proliferation.

Fluctuations in calcium ion release have been observed throughout the hydration process, with an initial reduction in calcium levels observed over the first 2–3 days, followed by an increase in calcium after 72 hours [41, 48]. There was no significant difference in calcium release between the two MTA color variants, but as demonstrated by several researchers, calcium elution and hydroxyapatite production were higher in the gray variant than the white one, both in the simulated tissue fluid solution and on the material's surface [24, 48]. As a result, the gray variant is expected to produce a better biological seal (sealing of voids, air bubbles, and capillary channels that may be present inadvertently in the material) than the white variant, preventing the penetration of bacteria and their toxins.

2.6 Synthetic Calcium Silicates

It is assumed that these materials are not produced by a clinkering of raw materials and are synthetic tricalcium silicate-based materials:

2.6.1 Biodentine

Biodentine is made up of tricalcium silicate, dicalcium silicate, calcium carbonate; zirconium oxide as a radio-opacifier; calcium oxide; iron oxide as a coloring agent and is mixed with a liquid that contains calcium chloride as a setting reaction accelerator; and a hydrosoluble polymer that acts as a water reducing agent. Biodentine has been reported to take a maximum of 45 minutes to set. Biodentine has a larger surface area than MTA. When compared to MTA-based cements, this results in faster hydration and set. The presence of heavy metal contaminants is thus expected to be reduced [49], but as previously stated, Biodentine contains arsenic and lead, but the release of these elements is low in simulated tissue fluid [31]. The main advantage of this material is that it has been used successfully as a temporary restoration with direct oral cavity exposure for up to six months [50]. This use, with direct oral cavity exposure, may be attributed to its higher compressive strength than comparable cements, or its calcium carbonate content, or the water-based mixing liquid containing calcium chloride and polycarboxylate [51–53]. This material has been referred to as the strongest dental calcium silicate cement, which was reported to reach as high as 300 MPa [34, 54].

2.6.2 BioAggregate

BioAggregate is a nanoparticulate material composed of tricalcium silicate, dicalcium silicate, calcium phosphate monobasic (hydroxyapatite), amorphous silicon oxide, and tantalum pentoxide as a radioopacifier. Deionized water is added to activate the hydration reaction. BioAggregates are devoid of aluminate, gypsum, and bismuth (III) oxide [55]. Calcium phosphates can strengthen bone cements and have been shown to stimulate the proliferation of human periodontal ligament fibroblasts [56]. The composition of BioAggregate is similar to that of the white variant of MTA, with the main differences being that it is fully synthetic, not derived from Portland cement, and free of aluminum [57]. Another distinction is the presence of calcium phosphate monobasic with the formula $Ca(H_2PO_4)_2$ and tantalum pentoxide. Therefore, BioAggregate's modified formula is an example of an improved calcium silicate cement and an evolution of the MTA formula [55].

2.6.3 EndoSequence

EndoSequence is another recently developed bioceramic material [58]. EndoSequence is made up of calcium silicates, zirconium oxide, tantalum oxide, calcium phosphate monobasic, and filling and thickening agents, according to the manufacturer. EndoSequence putty has an initial setting time of one hour, and the complete setting time is three to four hours [33]. It is manufactured as a premixed product in moldable putty and preloaded injectable paste to provide the clinician with a homogeneous and consistent material that sets in the presence of moisture. This material's main selling point is its uniform consistency during placement, which improves handling even in the presence of moisture. The large particle size of EndoSequence has a significant impact on the setting time [59], and it may play a role in the material surface's reaction to the external environment. The large particle size may facilitate the strong binding ability to positively changed ions from the surrounding environment.

2.6.4 iRoot BP Plus

EndoSequence and iRoot BP Plus have the same formula, which includes zirconium oxide, calcium silicates, tantalum oxide, calcium phosphate monobasic, and filler and thickening agents. However, iRoot BP Plus takes five to seven days to fully set, as opposed to EndoSequence which takes only a few hours [33]. Because calcium phosphate was included in the manufacturing process of iRoot BP Plus, the amount of phosphate that was found in this synthetic material was, as was to be expected, greater than that which was found in ProRoot MTA. In addition to this, the concentrations of chromium found in iRoot BP Plus were noticeably lower [60]. The main advantage of iRoot BP Plus is that it is thought to be a promising MTA alternative because of its nanomodified nature and ease of use, particularly after reports of its superiority in tissue repair and high-quality tertiary dentin formation began to surface [61, 62].

2.6.5 NeoMTA Plus

NeoMTA Plus is a new tricalcium silicate material that comes in a finer powder form and contains dicalcium silicate, calcium sulphate, silica, and tantalum oxide as a radiopacifying agent. This radiopacifying agent is combined with a water-based gel that gives the material good handling properties. The main advantage of this material is that the powder-to-gel mixing ratio can be adjusted to produce a thin or thick mixture, with both consistencies being reliable and predictable in various clinical applications [63]. When NeoMTA Plus is prepared with a putty consistency, the setting time is one hour; however, when it is used with a loose consistency, the setting time may take up to five hours [33]. In comparison to MTA, the release of calcium and hydroxyl ions was greater and lasted for a longer period of time. This difference can be attributed to the use of finer particle size and the application of an organic gel, both of which increased the porosity, water sorption, ion release, and solubility of the material [63].

2.6.6 BioRoot RCS

BioRoot RCS is a powdered material made of tricalcium silicate, zirconium oxide (opacifier), and povidone that is mixed with an aqueous solution of calcium chloride and polycarboxylate. The main advantage of this material is that it sets in less than four hours and is becoming popular as a sealer in single-cone or lateral condensation root fillings [64, 65].

BioRoot RCS demonstrated immediate calcium ion release that remained high for up to one month, indicating long-term activity when compared to MTA, which had its maximum calcium release over the first three days [63].

2.7 Technical Report

In this technical report, we describe an easy way to obtain hydroxyapatite by immersing a disk of gray Portland cement in serum-free media. This work strengthens the presented concepts mentioned above and demonstrates the ability of Portland cement-based materials to form hydroxyapatite in the presence of physiological fluids.

2.7.1 Methods

One gray Portland cement disk (Hanson Ribblesdale Works CEM I Portland Cement, EN 197-1 standard, UK) was prepared with a diameter of 5 cm and thickness of 2 cm using a plastic mold. The disk was placed in a container

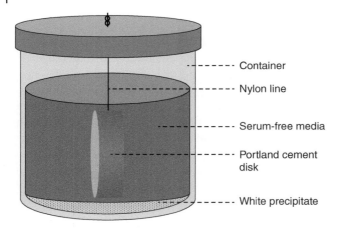

Container

Nylon line

Serum-free media

Portland cement disk

White precipitate

Figure 2.5 Illustration of the large material disk elution process.

containing 200 ml of serum-free media (D-MEM, Sigma Aldrich, Oakville, ON, Canada) and was incubated at 37 °C for two weeks (Figure 2.5). After the incubation period, the disk was removed and the white precipitate collected for further analysis using flame emission spectroscopy and X-ray diffraction.

2.7.1.1 Flame Emission Spectroscopy
The white precipitate was initially analyzed using flame emission spectroscopy to determine the presence of calcium in its structure.

Preparation of Standards
A stock solution of 10 mEq of calcium per liter was prepared by dissolving 0.5 g of $CaCO_3$ in 10 ml of concentrated HCl and diluting it to 1 l with distilled water.

Settings

Instrument:	Flame emission spectroscopy (Eppendorf ELEX 6361, Hamburg, Germany)
Oxygen:	22 inches of water pressure.
Gas:	Adjusted to give medium cones of blue flame, about 0.3–0.4 cm in height.
Air:	20 pounds per sq. in.
Wavelength:	The 556 rnp calcium oxide
Phototube:	The ultraviolet tube was used at 556 rnp
Slit width:	0.5 mm

2.7.1.2 X-ray Diffraction

The white powder was further analyzed using X-Ray diffraction. The powder was sintered to 1000 °C for 60 minutes. Sintering was performed to improve the particle size of the crystals for identification of its phase composition. The powder was milled with an agate mortar and pestle. X-ray diffraction patterns were recorded with a Shimadzu LabX XRD-6000 X-Ray diffractometer (Shimadzu, Japan). Results were analyzed by using the International Centre for Diffraction Data (ICDD) database [66].

Measurement Conditions

X-ray tube
Target = Cu
Voltage = 30 (kV)
Current = 30 (mA)

Slits
Divergence slit = 1.00000 (deg)
Scatter slit = 1.00000 (deg)
Receiving slit = 0.15000 (mm)

Scanning
Drive axis = Theta–2 Theta
Scan range = 20.000–50.000
Scan mode = Continuous scan
Scan speed = 2.0000 (deg/min)
Sampling pitch = 0.0200 (deg)
Preset time = 0.60 (s)

Procedure

The diffractometer used Cu radiation at 30 mA and 30 kV. The crystalline structure of the precipitate was determined by passing a beam of X-rays of known wavelength into the specimen while rotating it through an angle θ. The intensity of X-rays from the sample was measured by a detector. The detector was rotated between 20 and 50 at 0.02° θ per 0.6 second.

Phase identification was accomplished by use of search-match software utilizing ICDD database "previously known as the Joint Committee on Powder Diffraction Standards (JCPDS)." Diffraction patterns of known materials are documented in the powder diffraction files (PDF) found in the ICDD database.

In the ICDD card, the diffraction pattern of materials is indicated by the interplanar spacing "d," corresponding to each diffracted X-ray and the relative intensity of the diffracted X-ray.

The materials are represented by the value of the three strongest X-ray peaks and the relative intensity "I." The relative intensity indicates the quantity of a compound or constituent present in the material. After the experiment was run, the values of relative intensity "I" and theta angle "θ" were plotted. The proper group representing the strongest peak was located in the numerical index. Then the closest matches for the other two peaks were located and the relative intensities were compared with the tabulated values. When good agreement was found for all the three strongest lines, the proper data file was located and the relative intensities of all the lines were compared to complete the identification.

2.7.2 Results

The white precipitate collected from the gray Portland cement disk elute was found to have a weight of about 1.002 g after sintering (1000 °C for 60 minutes) (Figures 2.6 and 2.7). Initial analysis of the precipitated crystals using flame emission spectroscopy (Eppendorf ELEX 6361) showed that the percentage of calcium in the white precipitate was about 24%. Figure 2.8 shows the results of the X-ray diffraction analysis of the white precipitate. It can be seen that the crystals precipitated were chemically and structurally similar to the hydroxyapatite standard ICDD database, file 09-342) [66].

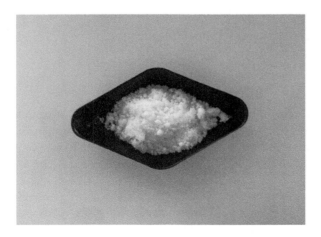

Figure 2.6 Precipitated hydroxyapatite.

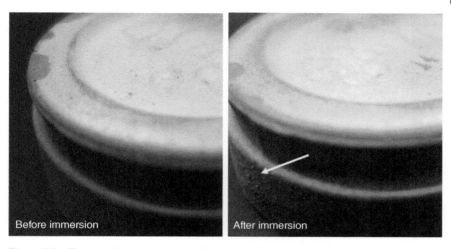

Before immersion

After immersion

Figure 2.7 The gray Portland cement disk surface before elution (left). The gray Portland cement disk surface after elution for two weeks (right). White precipitations are observed on its surface (arrow).

This technical report provides further evidence that Portland cement-based materials can form hydroxyapatite in the presence of phosphate-rich environments, supporting the previously presented insights.

2.8 Recommendations for Implementation

Endodontics is making increasing use of recently developed materials based on calcium silicate, which has led to an expansion of the application options available for these materials. It wasn't until 1993 [67] that calcium silicate-based materials were first mentioned in the scientific dental literature. Early research into calcium silicate-based materials' biological, physical, and chemical properties strongly highlighted the therapeutic potential of these materials. The unfavorable handling properties, prolonged setting time, potential for tooth and tissue staining, and high asking price have all contributed to the development of improved calcium silicate-based cements. These newer cements, according to their manufacturers, have fewer of these drawbacks.

The newer calcium silicate-based materials have been shown to be more biocompatible than their predecessors, which were either barely tolerated or severely cytotoxic. This has been reported numerous times in the literature, piquing the scientific community's interest in devising alternatives. As a result, both academic and commercial researchers have been motivated by the need to develop a

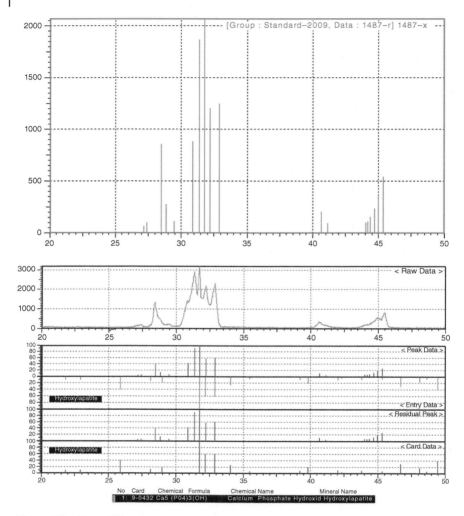

Figure 2.8 X-ray diffraction pattern obtained from gray Portland cement precipitate after sintering at 1000 C (top) and the comparison of patterns between the precipitate and hydroxyapatite standard (bottom).

restorative material with superior physical properties, enhanced user-friendliness, and improved biocompatibility.

In clinical practice, success is typically determined by the absence of symptoms, evidence of radiographic healing, and the patient's ability to continue using their tooth normally [68]. However, the absence of signs and symptoms and the radiographic appearance cannot truly demonstrate healing. The only method that can confirm true healing is histology, which is not an assessment method that can be used in everyday clinical practice.

Since their introduction in the 1990s, calcium silicate-based materials have undergone a radical transformation, and it's critical to realize that the scientific community now views this as a watershed moment in dental research that has greatly benefited both clinicians and patients. To be clear, none of this would have been possible without a plethora of meticulous studies, whether in the lab as in vitro experiments or clinical trials, which included numerous in situ, in vivo, and ex vivo trials. These studies provided researchers with invaluable information that helped them create the so-called "newer" calcium silicate-based materials that we are now seeing in development. It's also worth noting that the same methodology must be used whenever a new material is introduced, because the modifications and alterations in the original formula (i.e. Portland cement-based materials) need to be verified and subjected to the same tests that its predecessors have been subjected to. This is the reason why it is essential to take a step back and consider how the previous investigations into the older materials developed. This, in turn, can be of assistance to researchers in the verification, validation, and fine-tuning of new formulations that are currently being introduced into the dental market.

However, a large number of studies that compared different calcium silicate-based materials in vivo had a high risk of bias, low methodological quality, and high methodological heterogeneity [69]. The information that is gleaned from the emerging biological research on the subject of material characterization ought to be applied in the course of the planning and reporting of animal research in the field of endodontics. In spite of the fact that, over the course of the years, a variety of alternative calcium silicate-based materials have been developed; clinical trials on animal and human models have only been used to evaluate a few of these materials. Despite the methodological restrictions imposed on these studies, a comprehensive analysis of MTA was carried out and the results showed that the material in question exhibited the most predictable and appropriate biological behavior.

There are a number of research studies that in great detail describe the various chemical and physical characteristics of calcium silicate-based materials. On the other hand, it has been reported that an improvement in certain chemical and biological properties results in a negative effect on the physical parameters of the material in question [70]. Only a handful of studies have provided an in vivo examination of the newly developed materials by examining their effects on human teeth in clinical environments. The majority of research studies that have been published to this day are based on studies conducted in vitro on small laboratory animals. To find if new calcium silicate-based materials can be used in routine clinical settings, more clinical trials that compare MTA and the new calcium silicate-based materials need to be done.

2.9 Conclusion

We attempted to provide an up-to-date view of calcium silicate-based materials. MTA has been and continues to be the most important material. It currently dominates the global market owing to its ability to stimulate the deposition of hydroxyapatite on its surface and promote healing. The main constituents of new bioceramics continue to be heavily reliant on new calcium silicates. The synthetic materials hold great promise, but more research and development is needed to identify the ideal endodontic repair material.

A large number of new concepts and materials are still being researched. Some of them may result in significantly higher efficiency and lower costs in the coming decades. Calcium silicate-based materials still have a long way to go before they can make a revolutionary contribution to the dental profession, particularly endodontics. However, because so many different and promising materials and concepts have emerged since 1878, the chances of achieving this goal are good.

References

1 Dorozhkin, S. (2018). Current state of bioceramics. *Journal of Ceramic Science and Technology* 9 (4): 353–370.

2 Dorozhkin, S.V. (2010). Bioceramics of calcium orthophosphates. *Biomaterials* 31 (7): 1465–1485.

3 Parirokh, M. and Torabinejad, M. (2010). Mineral trioxide aggregate: a comprehensive literature review—part I: chemical, physical, and antibacterial properties. *Journal of Endodontia* 36 (1): 16–27.

4 Torabinejad, M. and Parirokh, M. (2010). Mineral trioxide aggregate: a comprehensive literature review—part II: leakage and biocompatibility investigations. *Journal of Endodontia* 36 (2): 190–202.

5 Parirokh, M. and Torabinejad, M. (2010). Mineral trioxide aggregate: a comprehensive literature review—part III: clinical applications, drawbacks, and mechanism of action. *Journal of Endodontia* 36 (3): 400–413.

6 Niu, L.-n., Jiao, K., Zhang, W. et al. (2014). A review of the bioactivity of hydraulic calcium silicate cements. *Journal of Dentistry* 42 (5): 517–533.

7 Srinath, P., Abdul Azeem, P., and Venugopal, R.K. (2020). Review on calcium silicate-based bioceramics in bone tissue engineering. *International Journal of Applied Ceramic Technology* 17 (5): 2450–2464.

8 Witte, D. (1878). The filling of a root canal with Portland cement. *German Quarterly for Dentistry* 18: 153–154.

9 Schlenker, M. (1880). Filling the root canals with Portland cement according to Dr Witte. *German Quarterly for Dentistry* 20: 277–283.

10 Nield, H. (2020). A short history of infection control in dentistry. *BDJ Team* 7 (8): 12–15.

11 Harlan, A.W. (1890). Why carbolic acid should be discarded by dentists. *The Dental Register* 45 (6): 302.

12 Torabinejad, M., Hong, C., McDonald, F., and Ford, T.P. (1995). Physical and chemical properties of a new root-end filling material. *Journal of Endodontics* 21 (7): 349–353.

13 Brophy, T.W. (1880). Carbolic acid and creasote—their chemistry and therapeutical application to the practice of dentistry. *The American Journal of Dental Science.* 14 (8): 348.

14 Torabinejad, M. and White, D.1995). Tooth filling material and method of use. United States Patent Office (June 23, 1998), Patent (5769638).

15 Bye, G.C. (1999). *Portland Cement: Composition, Production and Properties.* Thomas Telford.

16 Asgary, S., Parirokh, M., Eghbal, M.J., and Brink, F. (2004). A comparative study of white mineral trioxide aggregate and white Portland cements using X-ray microanalysis. *Australian Endodontic Journal* 30 (3): 89–92.

17 Funteas, U.R., Wallace, J., and Fochtman, F. (2003). A comparative analysis of mineral trioxide aggregate and Portland cement. *Australian Endodontic Journal* 29 (1): 43–44.

18 Asgary, S., Parirokh, M., Eghbal, M.J., and Brink, F. (2005). Chemical differences between white and gray mineral trioxide aggregate. *Journal of Endodontics* 31 (2): 101–103.

19 Camilleri, J., Montesin, F.E., Brady, K. et al. (2005). The constitution of mineral trioxide aggregate. *Dental Materials* 21 (4): 297–303.

20 Sarkar, N., Caicedo, R., Ritwik, P. et al. (2005). Physicochemical basis of the biologic properties of mineral trioxide aggregate. *Journal of Endodontics* 31 (2): 97–100.

21 Apaydin, E.S. and Torabinejad, M. (2004). The effect of calcium sulfate on hard-tissue healing after periradicular surgery. *Journal of Endodontics* 30 (1): 17–20.

22 Dental, D.T. (2002). ProRoot® MTA (mineral trioxide aggregate) root canal repair material. Material safety data. *Dentsply Tulsa Dental* 1–2.

23 Camilleri, J. and Pitt, F.T. (2006). Mineral trioxide aggregate: a review of the constituents and biological properties of the material. *International Endodontic Journal* 39 (10): 747–754.

24 Belío-Reyes, I.A., Bucio, L., and Cruz-Chavez, E. (2009). Phase composition of ProRoot mineral trioxide aggregate by X-ray powder diffraction. *Journal of Endodontics* 35 (6): 875–878.

25 Kahler, B. and Rossi-Fedele, G. (2016). A review of tooth discoloration after regenerative endodontic therapy. *Journal of Endodontics* 42 (4): 563–569.

26 Felman, D. and Parashos, P. (2013). Coronal tooth discoloration and white mineral trioxide aggregate. *Journal of Endodontics* 39 (4): 484–487.

27 Chang, S.W., Shon, W.J., Lee, W. et al. (2010). Analysis of heavy metal contents in gray and white MTA and 2 kinds of Portland cement: a preliminary study. *Oral Surgery, Oral Medicine, Oral Pathology, Oral Radiology, and Endodontology.* 109 (4): 642–646.

28 Primus, C.M. (2006). Comments on "Arsenic release provided by MTA and Portland cement" by Duarte MA, et al. *Oral Surgery, Oral Medicine, Oral Pathology, Oral Radiology and Endodontology.* 4 (101): 416–417.

29 Duarte, M.A.H., de Oliveira Demarchi, A.C.C., Yamashita, J.C. et al. (2005). Arsenic release provided by MTA and Portland cement. *Oral Surgery, Oral Medicine, Oral Pathology, Oral Radiology, and Endodontology.* 99 (5): 648–650.

30 Matsunaga, T., Tsujimoto, M., Kawashima, T. et al. (2010). Analysis of arsenic in gray and white mineral trioxide aggregates by using atomic absorption spectrometry. *Journal of Endodontics* 36 (12): 1988–1990.

31 Camilleri, J., Kralj, P., Veber, M., and Sinagra, E. (2012). Characterization and analyses of acid-extractable and leached trace elements in dental cements. *International Endodontic Journal* 45 (8): 737–743.

32 Tomljenovic, L. (2011). Aluminum and Alzheimer's disease: after a century of controversy, is there a plausible link? *Journal of Alzheimer's Disease* 23 (4): 567–598.

33 Parirokh, M., Torabinejad, M., and Dummer, P. (2018). Mineral trioxide aggregate and other bioactive endodontic cements: an updated overview–part I: vital pulp therapy. *International Endodontic Journal* 51 (2): 177–205.

34 Primus, C., Gutmann, J.L., Tay, F.R., and Fuks, A.B. (2022). Calcium silicate and calcium aluminate cements for dentistry reviewed. *Journal of the American Ceramic Society* 105 (3): 1841–1863.

35 Liu, W.-C., Wang, H.-Y., Chen, L.-C. et al. (2019). Hydroxyapatite/tricalcium silicate composites cement derived from novel two-step sol-gel process with good biocompatibility and applications as bone cement and potential coating materials. *Ceramics International* 45 (5): 5668–5679.

36 Islam, I., Chng, H.K., and Yap, A.U.J. (2006). Comparison of the physical and mechanical properties of MTA and Portland cement. *Journal of Endodontics* 32 (3): 193–197.

37 Komabayashi, T. and Spångberg, L.S. (2008). Comparative analysis of the particle size and shape of commercially available mineral trioxide aggregates and Portland cement: a study with a flow particle image analyzer. *Journal of Endodontics* 34 (1): 94–98.

38 Li, Q. and Coleman, N.J. (2015). The hydration chemistry of ProRoot MTA. *Dental Materials Journal* 34 (4): 458–465.

39 Asgary, S., Eghbal, M.J., Parirokh, M. et al. (2009). Comparison of mineral trioxide aggregate's composition with Portland cements and a new endodontic cement. *Journal of Endodontics* 35 (2): 243–250.

40 Turdean-Ionescu, C., Stevensson, B., Izquierdo-Barba, I. et al. (2016). Surface reactions of mesoporous bioactive glasses monitored by solid-state NMR: concentration effects in simulated body fluid. *The Journal of Physical Chemistry C.* 120 (9): 4961–4974.

41 Qutieshat, A.S., Al-Hiyasat, A.S., and Darmani, H. (2019). Biocompatibility evaluation of Jordanian Portland cement for potential future dental application. *Journal of Conservative Dentistry: JCD.* 22 (3): 249.

42 Tay, F.R., Pashley, D.H., Rueggeberg, F.A. et al. (2007). Calcium phosphate phase transformation produced by the interaction of the Portland cement component of white mineral trioxide aggregate with a phosphate-containing fluid. *Journal of Endodontics* 33 (11): 1347–1351.

43 Eanes, E.D. (2001). Amorphous calcium phosphate. *Monographs in Oral Science* 18: 130–147.

44 Meyer, J. and Eanes, E. (1978). A thermodynamic analysis of the amorphous to crystalline calcium phosphate transformation. *Calcified Tissue Research* 25 (1): 59–68.

45 Tanahashi, M., Kamiya, K., Suzuki, T., and Nasu, H. (1992). Fibrous hydroxyapatite grown in the gel system: effects of pH of the solution on the growth rate and morphology. *Journal of Materials Science. Materials in Medicine* 3 (1): 48–53.

46 LeGeros, R.Z. (1994). Biological and synthetic apatites. In: *Hydroxyapatite and Related Materials* (ed. P.W. Brown and B. Constantz), 3–28. Boca Raton, FL: CRC Press.

47 Sarkar, N., Saunders, B., Moiseyeva, R. et al. (ed.) (2002). Interaction of mineral trioside aggregate (MTA) with a synthetic tissue fluid. *Journal of Dental Research* 81 (Special Issue A): A–391.

48 Bozeman, T.B., Lemon, R.R., and Eleazer, P.D. (2006). Elemental analysis of crystal precipitate from gray and white MTA. *Journal of Endodontics* 32 (5): 425–428.

49 Camilleri, J., Sorrentino, F., and Damidot, D. (2013). Investigation of the hydration and bioactivity of radiopacified tricalcium silicate cement, Biodentine and MTA Angelus. *Dental Materials* 29 (5): 580–593.

50 Aggarwal, V., Singla, M., Yadav, S., and Yadav, H. (2015). Marginal adaptation evaluation of Biodentine and MTA Plus in "Open Sandwich" class II restorations. *Journal of Esthetic and Restorative Dentistry* 27 (3): 167–175.

51 PalatyŃska-Ulatowska, A., BuŁa, K., and Klimek, L. (2020). Influence of sodium hypochlorite and ultrasounds on surface features and chemical composition of Biodentine tricalcium silicate-based material. *Dental Materials Journal* 39: 587–592.

52 Govindaraju, L., Neelakantan, P., and Gutmann, J.L. (2017). Effect of root canal irrigating solutions on the compressive strength of tricalcium silicate cements. *Clinical Oral Investigations* 21 (2): 567–571.

53 Kayahan, M.B., Nekoofar, M.H., McCann, A. et al. (2013). Effect of acid etching procedures on the compressive strength of 4 calcium silicate–based endodontic cements. *Journal of Endodontics* 39 (12): 1646–1648.

54 Butt, N., Talwar, S., Chaudhry, S. et al. (2014). Comparison of physical and mechanical properties of mineral trioxide aggregate and Biodentine. *Indian Journal of Dental Research* 25 (6): 692.

55 Park, J.-W., Hong, S.-H., Kim, J.-H. et al. (2010). X-ray diffraction analysis of white ProRoot MTA and Diadent BioAggregate. *Oral Surgery, Oral Medicine, Oral Pathology, Oral Radiology, and Endodontology.* 109 (1): 155–158.

56 Kasaj, A., Willershausen, B., Reichert, C. et al. (2008). Ability of nanocrystalline hydroxyapatite paste to promote human periodontal ligament cell proliferation. *Journal of Oral Science* 50 (3): 279–285.

57 De-Deus, G., Canabarro, A., Alves, G. et al. (2009). Optimal cytocompatibility of a bioceramic nanoparticulate cement in primary human mesenchymal cells. *Journal of Endodontics* 35 (10): 1387–1390.

58 Damas, B.A., Wheater, M.A., Bringas, J.S., and Hoen, M.M. (2011). Cytotoxicity comparison of mineral trioxide aggregates and EndoSequence bioceramic root repair materials. *Journal of Endodontics* 37 (3): 372–375.

59 Ha, W.N., Bentz, D.P., Kahler, B., and Walsh, L.J. (2015). D90: the strongest contributor to setting time in mineral trioxide aggregate and Portland cement. *Journal of Endodontics* 41 (7): 1146–1150.

60 Tian, J., Zhang, Y., Lai, Z. et al. (2017). Ion release, microstructural, and biological properties of iRoot BP Plus and ProRoot MTA exposed to an acidic environment. *Journal of Endodontics* 43 (1): 163–168.

61 Okamoto, M., Takahashi, Y., Komichi, S. et al. (2018). Novel evaluation method of dentin repair by direct pulp capping using high-resolution micro-computed tomography. *Clinical Oral Investigations* 22 (8): 2879–2887.

62 Shi, S., Bao, Z., Liu, Y. et al. (2016). Comparison of in vivo dental pulp responses to capping with iR oot BP Plus and mineral trioxide aggregate. *International Endodontic Journal* 49 (2): 154–160.

63 Siboni, F., Taddei, P., Prati, C., and Gandolfi, M. (2017). Properties of Neo MTA Plus and MTA Plus cements for endodontics. *International Endodontic Journal* 50: e83–e94.

64 Siboni, F., Taddei, P., Zamparini, F. et al. (2017). Properties of BioRoot RCS, a tricalcium silicate endodontic sealer modified with povidone and polycarboxylate. *International Endodontic Journal* 50:e120–e136.

65 Simon, S. and Flouriot, A.-C. (2016). BioRoot™ RCS a new biomaterial for root canal filling. *Journal of Case Studies Collection.* 13: 4–11.

66 Hubbard, C. and O'Connor, B. (2002). International centre for diffraction data (ICDD). *The National Conference and Exhibition of the Australian X-ray Analytical Association Inc. INIS 34 (21). Analytical X-ray for Industry and Science*, Newcastle.

67 Lee, S.-J., Monsef, M., and Torabinejad, M. (1993). Sealing ability of a mineral trioxide aggregate for repair of lateral root perforations. *Journal of Endodontics* 19 (11): 541–544.

68 Johnson, B.R. (1999). Considerations in the selection of a root-end filling material. *Oral Surgery, Oral Medicine, Oral Pathology, Oral Radiology, and Endodontology.* 87 (4): 398–404.

69 Pinheiro, L.S., Kopper, P.M.P., Quintana, R.M. et al. (2021). Does MTA provide a more favourable histological response than other materials in the repair of furcal perforations? A systematic review. *International Endodontic Journal* 54 (12): 2195–2218.

70 Palczewska-Komsa, M., Kaczor-Wiankowska, K., and Nowicka, A. (2021). New bioactive calcium silicate cement ineral Trioxide Aggregate Repair High Plasticity (MTA HP)—a systematic review. *Material* 14 (16): 4573.

3

Bioceramics in Clinical Endodontics

Ayfer Atav[1], Burçin Arıcan[2], and Keziban Olcay[3]

[1] *Faculty of Dentistry, Department of Endodontics, Istinye University, Istanbul, Turkey*
[2] *School of Dental Medicine, Department of Endodontics, Bahçeşehir University, Istanbul, Turkey*
[3] *Faculty of Dentistry, Department of Endodontics, Istanbul University-Cerrahpaşa, Istanbul, Turkey*

CONTENTS

Bioceramics in Endodontics, First Edition. Edited by Viresh Chopra.
© 2024 John Wiley & Sons, Inc. Published 2024 by John Wiley & Sons, Inc.
Companion website: www.wiley.com/go/chopra/bioceramicsinendodontics

3.1   Introduction

In recent years, there have been many developments in the practice of endodontics. The most promising among them is bioceramics, which provides ease of use in all areas, from vital pulp therapy to routine root canal treatments and from regeneration cases to apical surgery.

In fact, the history of hydraulic cements begins with the Roman Empire. The Romans used this water and cement mixture in all their infrastructure works. However, the patent of today's known Portland cement could only be obtained in the nineteenth century. The use of hydraulic cement in the dental field ranges from Portland cement, which initiates the hydration reaction, to mineral trioxide aggregate (MTA) and then to tricalcium silicate-based bioceramic materials [1].

The precursor of today's bioceramic materials was calcium phosphate root canal sealers such as Sankin and Capseal which were described in 1984 [2, 3]. The first step of today's bioceramic materials was taken in the mid-1990s with MTA produced from Portland cement. The first product introduced in the market is ProRoot MTA (Dentsply Tulsa Dental, Tulsa, OK, USA) which has been released as root repair material and pulp capping material [4]. Then, bioceramic-based root canal sealers took a place in endodontic practice. BioAggregate (Innovative Bioceramix, Vancouver, BC, Canada), which has calcium silicate as a main component instead of Portland cement, offered a new breath to the endodontics in the beginning of the 2000s [5]. Today, these calcium-based materials ensure better endodontic therapies with their features such as biocompatibility, high alkaline pH, bioactivity, hydrophilic structure, high sealing ability, dimensional stability, and fracture resistance [6].

In this chapter, the physicochemical properties, biological properties, preparation methods, and usage areas of bioceramic-based materials on the market will be examined in detail from past to present.

3.2 Classification of Hydraulic Cements in Endodontics

Hydraulic cements can be classified according to their chemistry (Table 3.1), their use in endodontics (Table 3.2) [7], or their major components [3]. Considering the chemistry, all the hydraulic cements have four main components. These are cement, radiopacifer, vehicle, and additives. While the main component of Type 1, Type 2, and Type 3 cements are Portland cement, Type 4 and Type 5 cements are tricalcium silicate-based [7]. These classifications will help the clinicians understand the ingredients and their application areas.

3.2.1 Type 1 Hydraulic Cements

3.2.1.1 ProRoot MTA

ProRoot MTA (Dentsply Tulsa Dental, Tulsa, OK, USA) (Figure 3.1) is the first primitive form of bioceramics and was produced in 1993. Then, the white and tooth-colored forms were manufactured in 2002. Principal components of the material are tricalcium silicate, dicalcium silicate, bismuth oxide, and calcium sulfate. Bismuth oxide is the radiopacifier inside the material and the possible responsible ingredient for the discoloration [8]. Its liquid is 100% distilled water. It has high radiopacity (6.47 mm aluminum [Al]) [4].

It has been used in endodontics for its low cytotoxicity, biocompatibility, and osteogenetic and cementogenetic features [9, 10]. It complies with ISO standards (ISO 9917) [9]. Setting time is three to four hours [8]. It has a better adaptation to dentine when compared to formerly used materials like amalgam [11]. On the other hand, it should be applied at least 3 mm to increase the sealing and adherence ability during apical surgery applications or root repair. The origin of the adaptation comes from the hydroxyapatite crystals that appear in the product's consequent series of reactions [11]. It can be used for pulp capping, apexification, root-end filling, perforation and resorption repair [4]. Kim et al. [12] observed that the use of MTA in pulp capping created in an inflammatory environment reduced the inflammation. Although it has excellent features, the tough handling and long setting time still constitute some problems in clinical applications [13].

Table 3.1 Classification of hydraulic cements based on chemistry.

Type	Cement	Radiopacifer	Additive	Water	Brand name
1	Portland cement	+/−	−	+	ProRoot MTA
2	Portland cement	+	+	+	MTA Angelus MM-MTA MTA-HP
3	Portland cement	+	+	−	EndoSeal MTA Fillapex TheraCal PT TheraCal LC
4	Tricalcium/ dicalcium silicate	+	+	+	BioAggregate Biodentine BioRoot RCS MTA Bioseal Bio-C Pulpo MTA Repair HP
5	Tricalcium/ dicalcium silicate	+	+	−	Total Fill® TotalFill® BC Sealer HiFlow™ TotalFill® BC RRM TotalFill® BC RRM™ Putty TotalFill® BC RRM™ Fast set Putty iRoot SP iRoot BP iRoot BP Plus iRoot FS EndoSequence® BC Sealer EndoSequence® BC Sealer HiFlow EndoSequence® BC Root Repair material (ERRM) EndoSequence® BC RRM Putty EndoSequence® BC RRM Fast set Puty Bioceramic Root Repair Material (BC RRM) Well-Root ST CeraSeal MTA Bioseal Bio-C Repair Bio-C Sealer Bio-C Temp Bio-C Pulpecto Bio-C Sealer ION+ AH Plus Bioceramic Sealer

Source: Camilleri [7]/Springer Nature.

Table 3.2 Classification of hydraulic cements based on their specific use in endodontology [7].

Location	Specific use	Brand name
Intracoronal	Pulp capping materials Regenerative endodontic cements	All Type 4 hydraulic cements (Table 3.1) and MTA
Intraradicular	Root canal sealer Apical plug cements	Biodentine MTA MTA BioSeal BioRoot RCS TotalFill® BC sealer TotalFill® BC sealer Hiflow TotalFill® BC RRM EndoSequence® BC EndoSequence® BC HiFlow EndoSequence® BC RRM EndoSequence® BC RRM fast set putty iRoot SP iRoot BP iRoot BP Plus iRoot FS MTA BIOREP Well Root ST Bio-C CeraSeal BioRoot RCS
Extraradicular	Root-end filling materials Perforation repair cements	Biodentine MTA TotalFill® BC putty EndoSequence® BC putty iRoot BP Plus MTA BIOREP

Source: Camilleri [7]/Springer Nature.

3.2.2 Type 2 Hydraulic Cements

Type 2 hydraulic cements are Portland-based cements. Most of them have additives for improving some mechanical, physical, or biological properties of the materials [7].

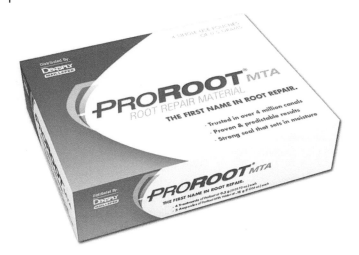

Figure 3.1 ProRoot MTA. *Source:* Dental World Official.

3.2.2.1 MTA Angelus

MTA Angelus (Angelus, Londrina, Brazil) is bioceramic regenerative cement containing MTA. It was launched in 2001 in two forms, gray and white [14]. It is boxed as powder and liquid in a bottle which is easier than ProRoot MTA to store for reuse. The powder contains 80% Portland cement and 20% bismuth oxide [15]. Its liquid is distilled water. Each box contains five 1 g bottles and a 3 ml liquid bottle.

MTA Angelus has an initial curing time of 10 minutes and a final setting time of 15 minutes. It was reported that it can be a good option in clinical use because of its short setting time [16]. Owing to its lower bismuth oxide content, it shows less radiopacity than ProRoot MTA [17]. Its marginal adaptation was found to be lower than MTA [18].

Some additives such as calcium oxide in its contents are aimed at enhancing the early release of calcium hydroxide [19]. The early release of these calcium ions accelerates dentine bridge formation and biological healing after pulp capping. It also provides biological repair of perforations and injured periradicular tissues. Calcium sulfate in its content has been removed to reduce the setting time [20]. It is biologically compatible and does not show cytotoxic and mutagenic properties [21–23]. In addition, according to the results of some studies, MTA Angelus has antimicrobial properties [15, 16, 20].

Its content allows it to be used under moist conditions. Therefore, it is easy to use and has wide indications in endodontic practice such as perforations, apexification, internal resorption, pulpotomy, pulp exposure, root-end fillings, apexification, and apexogenesis [19].

3.2.2.2 MTA Bio

MTA Bio (Angelus Ind. Prod., Londrina, Brazil) is a water-based Portland cement synthesized under highly controlled laboratory conditions and developed to prevent the presence of arsenic and lead in cement dust [24]. It is known that its content consists of 80% Portland cement and 20% bismuth oxide [25]. The manufacturer reports that the final cement is free of unwanted contaminants, especially arsenic [26].

It sets completely in two hours [27]. The radiopacity of MTA Bio was found to comply with the 3 mm Al radiopacity [27]. Owing to its low solubility and high purity, it shows low cytotoxicity on odontoblast-like cells [28]. It has been reported that it is more effective in wound healing and accelerates healing after pulp capping or pulpotomy [28].

3.2.2.3 MM-MTA™

MM-MTA™ (Micro-Mega Besancon, France) (Figure 3.2) is water-insoluble endodontic repair cement. It was developed in 2011 [29]. The content is as follows: tricalcium silicate, bismuth oxide, tricalcium aluminate, magnesium oxide,

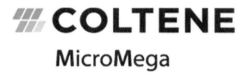

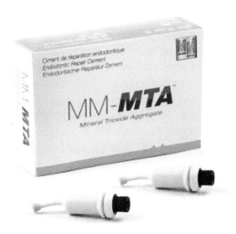

Figure 3.2 MM-MTA. *Source:* COLTENE Group.

calcium sulfate dihydrate, calcium carbonate ($CaCO_3$), and chloride accelerator [30]. MM-MTA™ consists of powder and liquid capsules. Its powder consists of very fine hydraulic particles of several mineral oxides. It is mixed automatically with a vibrating mixer. Thus, powder and liquid are always mixed in the right proportion, and homogeneity of the material can be achieved [31].

It has been reported that the working time of MM-MTA™ is approximately 2 minutes (at 23 °C) and the setting time is 20 minutes [32]. The short setting time is related to the calcium carbonate and chloride accelerator content [33]. Also, calcium carbonate makes the manipulation of MM-MTA™ easier [30]. Its radiopacity is similar to that of MTA.

It has been shown that MM-MTA™ is safe to use because it contains acceptable levels of arsenic, lead, and metal oxides [34]. It is biocompatible and has excellent adhesion to dentine [30]. MM-MTA™ was shown to support odontologic [35] and osteogenic differentiation stem cells [36].

3.2.3 Type 3 Hydraulic Cements

Type 3 hydraulic cements are also Portland cements. Alternative vehicles are used instead of water in Type 3 cements.

3.2.3.1 EndoSeal MTA

EndoSeal MTA (Maruchi, Wonju, Korea) (Figure 3.3a) is a ready-to-use, injectable, pozzolan-based root canal sealer. Thanks to its high fluidity, it could be used with the single-cone technique [37, 38]. It has ingredients similar to the MTA, such as calcium silicates, calcium aluminates, calcium aluminoferrite, calcium sulfates, radiopacifier, and a thickening agent [39].

EndoSeal MTA absorbs the ambient moisture in the root canal throughout the setting reaction [40]. It completes its self-curing and no mixing is required [41]. Therefore, it is less technique sensitive. Its setting time has been reported as 12.31 minutes [39]. In a review of calcium silicate-based-sealers, it was reported that EndoSeal MTA has similar solubility, lower radiopacity, and higher alkalinity and fluidity compared to AH Plus sealer [42].

It has been indicated that EndoSeal MTA has the good sealing ability, dimensional stability, insolubility, and optimal biocompatibility [41, 43]. It also provides satisfactory and favorable biological and physicochemical properties [44] It has good bond strength to dentine, high fracture resistance [45], low discoloration [39, 46], and superior sealer distribution [47]. Also, its alkalinity level is similar to MTA [41]. Recent studies reported that the antibacterial activity of EndoSeal MTA is highly effective [48], and comparable to that of ProRoot MTA [49].

3.2.3.2 MTA Fillapex

MTA Fillapex (Angelus, Londrina, PR, Brazil) (Figure 3.3d) is a disalicylate resin-based endodontic sealer that contains 40% MTA particles [50]. It was introduced

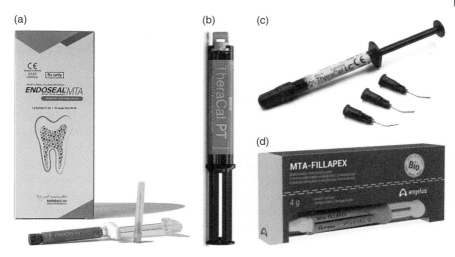

Figure 3.3 Some Type 3 Hydraulic cement in the market. (a) EndoSeal MTA. (b) Theracal PT. (c) Theracal LC. (d) MTA Fillapex.

commercially in 2010 with a high sealing capacity and ability to promote cementum regeneration [51]. According to the manufacturer, its ingredients are as follows (Paste A and Paste B, respectively): salicylate resin for ionic polymer formation, bismuth trioxide for radiopacity, fumed silica as filler, 40% MTA as active ingredient and responsible for ionic polymer formation, base resin for plasticity, fumed silica as filler and titanium dioxide as pigment. It is ready to use [52]. The material has excellent calcium ion release, biocompatibility, excellent flow, and easy removal. Despite that, it has also been reported that it releases less calcium ions than MTA and that no calcium hydroxide is detected during its hydration [53].

It was stated that the setting time of the material was 19.3 minutes and the failure of the material setting procedure was observed in dry conditions [39].

Contrary to the manufacturer's instructions [52] and some studies, there are also studies stating that MTA Fillapex is highly cytotoxic [54] and induces a long-term inflammatory reaction [55]. It has been demonstrated that the cytotoxicity of MTA Fillapex may be due to its alkaline pH [56], high dissolution rate [57] or incapability in releasing ions required for apatite formation [58], and entity of resin in the MTA-Fillapex's structure [59].

3.2.3.3 TheraCal LC

TheraCal LC (Bisco Inc, Schaumburg, IL, USA) (Figure 3.3c) which is a light-curing, resin-modified, Portland cement-based filled liner developed in 2011. It is aimed to be used as a protective base under restorative materials in direct and indirect pulp capping therapies. It is used for the protection and isolation of the dental pulpal complex. It is composed of 45% type III Portland cement, 40% resin, 10% barium sulfate for radiopacity, and 5% fumed silica [60].

The product does not need mixing. It is packaged and ready to use in a syringe.

According to the manufacturer, the tricalcium silicate particles in the hydrophilic resin matrix of the TheraCal LC provide a significant calcium ion release (213 (μg/cm^2)/24 h). The ion release stimulates hydroxyapatite and the dentine bridge formation provides a tight seal and makes the material uniquely stable. It is stated by the manufacturer that its alkaline pH (10–11 in three hours) can promote healing, pulpal vitality, and apatite formation. In addition, due to the light-curing structure of the material, it allows the restorative material to be placed immediately, providing easy handling usage for the clinician. It has 2.6 mm Al radiopacity. TheraCal LC can be used with all etch techniques (self-selective and total-etch) for optimal bonding of the restoration. It is moisture tolerant and will not wash out or dissolve over time. In a recently published meta-analysis, it was stated that the bond strength of TheraCal LC to resin composite materials is better when using a total-etch adhesive system [61]. The manufacturer recommends light-curing each 1 mm cement for 20 seconds [62].

3.2.3.4 TheraCal PT

TheraCal PT (Bisco, Inc., Schaumburg, IL, USA) (Figure 3.3b) is a new, resin-modified Portland-based material. It is dual-cured. It has been marketed in a syringe and is ready to use. According to the manufacturer, it is primarily indicated for pulpotomy, and it may also be used for direct (pulp exposures) and indirect (protective liner) vital pulp therapies. The chemical formulation of TheraCal PT is similar to TheraCal LC and contains synthetic Portland cement and calcium silicate particles in a hydrophilic matrix. It has been stated that this structure facilitates calcium release [63].

The manufacturer of the product claimed that its pH is 11.5 at seven days; it presents low water solubility and has 2.45 mm Al radiopacity. It is reported by the manufacturer that TheraCal PT has minimum 45 seconds of working time at 35 °C and maximum of 5 minutes of setting time at 35 °C. This allows the treatment to be completed in a single session [63].

In recent studies carried out to test the bioactive properties of the material, TheraCal PT was found to be less cytotoxic than TheraCal LC [64], and TheraCal PT exhibited similar biological results as MTA Angelus [64], and Biodentine [65]. Another recently published study noted that TheraCal PT exhibited limited bioactivity [66]. However, more in vitro, in vivo, and clinical studies are needed for TheraCal PT.

3.2.4 Type 4 Hydraulic Cements

Type 4 hydraulic cements are tricalcium silicate-based. They are not premixed; in other words, not ready to use. The powder is mixed with a liquid. The main idea behind creating Type 4 hydraulic cements is the difficult use of MTA because of its long setting time, cost, discoloration problem, and difficulties in handling procedure.

3.2.4.1 BioAggregate

BioAggregate (Innovative Bioceramix, Vancouver, BC, Canada) is a novel laboratory-synthesized water-based cement [67]. It was patented in 2006 [68], but introduced as a product in 2008. The first product where the definition of bioceramic is mentioned is BioAggragate [68]. It is an improved form of white MTA. It contains tricalcium silicate, dicalcium silicate, silicon dioxide, tantalum peroxide, calcium phosphate, and phosphorus [69]. But differently from white MTA, it is aluminum-free and contains calcium phosphate monobasic, and tantalum pentoxide. While the former adjusts its hydrate setting, the latter works as a radiopacifer [70]. BioAggregate powder which contains bioceramic nanoparticles is mixed with BioA Liquid (deionized water) (Figure 3.4a) [5].

According to the manufacturer's claims, it is a biocompatible material because of its aluminum-free construction. Its working time is reported as at least 5 minutes. The mixture of powder and liquid composes a thick paste-like structure which makes manipulation easier. Since all the materials in its contents are white, the color obtained after mixing adapts to the natural tooth color [5]. Because of the lack of bismuth oxide, no tooth discoloration is expected [69]. The radiopacity of BioAggregate is equal to 3.8 mm Al, meeting ISO standards [71].

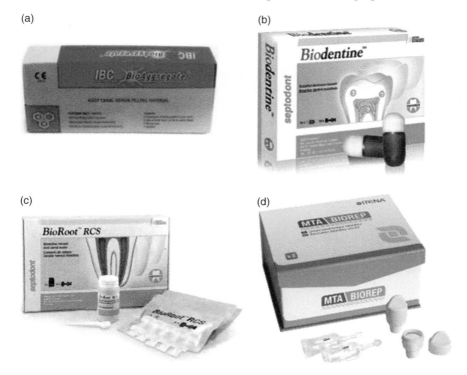

(a)

(b)

(c)

(d)

Figure 3.4 Type 4 hydraulic cements in the market. *Sources:* (a) LocalDentist.pro / https://localdentist.pro/dental-root-canal-filling-material/ (accessed 9 May 2023). (b, c) Septodont Holding. (d) Itena Clinical.

BioAggregate is insoluble in tissue fluids and has antimicrobial features [72]. It is a nontoxic and biocompatible material which is shown by the deposition of hydroxyapatite [73]. When hydrated, tricalcium silicate produces calcium silicate hydrate and calcium hydroxide. Its calcium ion release is quite high and sustains it over a 28-day period [69]. Mineralization, odontoblastic differentiation effect on human dental pulp cells, and antimicrobial activity against Enterococcus faecalis is comparable to MTA [73, 74]. Also, it showed similar cell viability with MTA [73] and Biodentine [74]. Its strength against acid is more than MTA [75]. On the other hand, its push-out bond strength was reported lower than MTA and common failure mode was shown as cohesive [76].

3.2.4.2 Biodentine™

Biodentine™ (Septodont, Saint-Maur-des-Fosses, France) was released to the market in the beginning of 2009 by Septodont. It is developed with Active Biosilicate Technology™, which can purify the calcium silicate content by depriving it of aluminate and calcium silicate [77]. It is marketing in capsule/liquid form which ensures an easier clinical application (Figure 3.4b). This specific ratio allows the clinician to use optimally prepared material every time. The powder of Biodentine mainly contains tricalcium silicate ($3Cao\,SiO_2$) as the main core material and calcium carbonate ($CaCO_3$) as a filler. It also contains dicalcium silicate (second core material), iron oxide, and zirconium oxide which is responsible for the material's radiopacity. The liquid of the material contains calcium chloride as an accelerator and hydrosoluble polymer as a water reducing agent. The powder in the capsule is mixed with the liquid for 30 seconds with a triturator at 4000–4200 rpm [78].

Biodentine mainly has superior physicochemical properties. The working time is about 1 minute and the setting time is between 9 and 12 minutes because of the calcium chloride in the liquid [79]. According to Grech et al. [80], these values only show the initial setting time and the final setting time can be up to 45 minutes. Thanks to its zirconium oxide content, it displays a radiopacity equivalent to 3.5 mm of aluminum which is over the minimum requirement of ISO standards [77].

The porosity of the material affects the amount of microleakage. Therefore, it is a very important factor that should be taken into consideration, especially in vital pulp treatments and regeneration procedures. Camilleri et al. [19] tested Biodentine both in a dry environment and immersed in a physiological solution. The results showed that microcracks and gaps were observed on the surface of Biodentine in dry conditions. However, lesser porosity was determined in the moisture environment [19]. Given this situation, it is important to consider the use of Biodentine in certain clinical situations.

In the literature, the Vickers microhardness value of Biodentine varies between 51 and 130 HV [19]. Considering the Vickers microhardness value of intact dentine varies between 60 and 90 HV [81], it could be concluded that Biodentine has similar mechanical behavior to human sound dentine.

According to the manufacturer's reports, the resistance of Biodentine to the acidic environment is limited. However, in the phosphate-containing saliva medium, Biodentine reportedly showed crystal deposition on its surface, which the company calls an "apatite-like" structure, which may increase the material's marginal sealing ability [77].

In the biologic aspect, Biodentine is a non-genotoxic, bioactive, and biocompatible material [82]. It was shown that when Biodentine had direct contact with pulp, it induced proliferation, migration and adhesion of human dental pulp stem cells [83]. Besides this, it also has antimicrobial properties thanks to its high alkaline pH. It can induce odontoblastic differentiation and stimulate dentine bridge formation. Therefore, it can be used safely as a pulp capping material [84].

Biodentine has a wide range of applications in restorative, endodontics, and pedodontics practice. It is the only material in the market that can be used as a temporary enamel substitute up to six months [79] and permanent dentine restorations such as deep/large carious lesions, deep cervical/radicular lesions, indirect pulp capping, direct pulp capping, pulpotomy, and partially pulpotomy. Beside it can be used in several areas on root surfaces such as perforations, external or internal resorptions, regenerative endodontics, apexogenesis, apexification, and as retrograde filling material [77].

3.2.4.3 BioRoot RCS

BioRoot root canal sealer (BioRoot RCS; Septodont, Saint-Maur-des-Fosses, France), which has been based on the background of Biodentine, has been in the market as a root canal sealer since the beginning of the first quarter of 2015 [85]. It has been developed in powder and liquid form (Figure 3.4c). The powder contains tricalcium silicate, zirconium oxide (opacifier), and povidone, while the liquid is composed of calcium chlorite and polycarboxylate [86]. BioRoot RCS is prepared by mixing 1/5 (powder/liquid) with a spoon for 60 seconds [87].

According to the manufacturer's information, its radiopacity is more than 5 mm aluminum. It is recommended to use with single cone or cold lateral condensation technique. Its pH value is more than 11 and final setting time is 240 minutes [87]. It was reported that the push-out bond strength was lower than AH Plus, and EDTA solution negatively affected this strength [88].

Several researches showed that BioRoot RCS has antimicrobial [89] and antibacterial activity because of its high alkaline pH [86]. Considering the studies showing that high Ca^{+2} ion release plays a key role in endodontic regeneration [90], BioRoot RCS, which has been shown to prolong the release of calcium ions, is considered to be bioactive and biocompatible [86]. Jeanneau et al. [91] reported that BioRoot RCS has anti-inflammatory effects and stimulates tissue regeneration initiated by human periodontal ligament fibroblast. Similarly, its antibacterial activity against E. faecalis was revealed as higher than TotalFill® BC and AH Plus sealer [92].

3.2.4.4 MTA BIOREP

MTA BIOREP (Itena, Villepinte, France) is a high-plasticity endodontic bioceramic restorative cement. It is marketed in capsule and liquid form (Figure 3.4d). The powder is composed of tricalcium silicate, dicalcium silicate, tricalcium aluminate, calcium oxide, and calcium tungstate. The liquid includes distilled water and activating agent [93]. The powder and liquid can be mixed by using a spatula, an amalgam holder, or an MTA gun carrier type device. In the product sheet, it is recommended to pour four drops of liquid into the powder cap and shake for 30 seconds on a mixing device [93].

According to the manufacturer's claims, it has superior features, such as fast setting time (15 minutes), easy manipulation, excellent marginal sealing ability, and lower solubility, when compared with other similar products on the market [94]. Its pH value is 9.3. The radiopacity is 3.7 mm of Al. MTA BIOREP indications are reported to be direct pulp capping, pulpotomy, internal resorption, apexification, apexogenesis, furcation, and root canal perforation [94]. There is no study in the literature that investigates the physicochemical and biological features of this product, yet.

3.2.4.5 Bio-C Pulpo

A calcium silicate-based bioceramic material Bio-C Pulpo (Angelus, Londrina, Paraná, Brazil) has recently been produced to improve some of the difficulties and undesirable situations found in other materials on the market. Its ingredients are tricalcium silicate, dicalcium silicate, calcium hydroxide, silicon dioxide, calcium fluoride, calcium aluminate, zirconium oxide, and iron oxide in powder, and distilled water, calcium chloride, methylparaben, and plasticizing material in liquid [95]. Calcium hydroxide and silicon dioxide with zirconium oxide used as a radiopacifier in the powder; calcium chloride and methylparaben are used as plasticizing material in the mixing liquid. Bio-C Pulpo's most appropriate clinical use is pulpotomy. According to the manufacturer, it is also indicated as a cavity liner in atraumatic restorative treatment. In addition, this material allows the restorative procedure to be performed in the same session [96].

Bio-C Pulpo is a biocompatible material and studies showed that it performed with similar mineralization capacity to MTA and similar induction of some osteogenic markers to MTA Angelus [95]. In other studies comparing Bio-C Pulpo, MTA Repair HP, and MTA Angelus, all materials were found to be biocompatible [96]. However, Bio-C Pulpo was the material with the highest cytotoxicity [96], and induced more inflammatory reaction than other materials [97]. However, these results need to be supported by other studies.

3.2.4.6   MTA Repair HP

MTA Repair HP (Angelus, Londrina, PR, Brazil) has been developed as a bioceramic high-plasticity reparative material with a shorter setting time (15 minutes) and improved handling properties to overcome some chemical and physical difficulties related to MTA [98]. Its composition includes tricalcium silicate, tricalcium aluminate, calcium oxide, dicalcium silicate, and calcium tungstate as powder; water and plasticizer as liquid [99]. Each box is packed as 10 capsules of powder, each 0.085 g and 10 bottles of liquid. Its mixing ratio: 0.085 g of powder (1 package) and 0.25 g of liquid (1 drop) [98].

Its radiopacity is greater than 3 mm Al and its solubility is 0.005% [98]. MTA Repair HP is indicated for root and furcation perforations, internal resorption, surgical treatment of root perforation, retrofilling, pulp capping, pulpotomy, apexogenesis, and apexification [98].

Its structure is based on the structure of MTA [100]. Unlike conventional MTA preparations, MTA Repair HP includes calcium tungstate instead of bismuth oxide as radiopacifier and a mixing liquid instead of distilled water as a plasticizer agent [98]. It is stated that calcium tungstate usage improves the physicochemical characteristics and handling properties of MTA Repair HP and it also prevents tooth staining [101]. In addition, calcium tungstate has been shown to be more biocompatible than bismuth oxide [102]. It is known that the presence of a plasticizer agent in the mixing liquid provides higher plasticity and improved handling characteristics to the material [100]. The researchers indicated that the calcium tungstate usage in MTA Repair HP causes higher calcium release at the first phases and improves the biomineralization process and the resistance of the material [103]. This increases the biomechanical properties of the material and provides greater flowability [100].

3.2.5   Type 5 Hydraulic Cements

Type 5 hydraulic cements are tricalcium silicate-based materials. They do not include water. They are premixed and ready to use.

3.2.5.1   iRoot SP, EndoSequence® BC, TotalFill®

iRoot SP (Innovative BioCeramix, Inc., Vancouver, Canada) was one of the first produced tricalcium-based bioceramic sealers in 2007 [88]. This product can be found in the market with the same content and different brands as EndoSequence®

BC (Brasseler, Savannah AU, USA) and TotalFill® (FKG, La Chaux- de-Fonds, Switzerland) (Figure 3.5a) [7]. They are identical and their compositions are zirconium oxide, dicalcium silicate, tricalcium silicate, calcium phosphate monobasic, calcium hydroxide, filler, and thickening agents [104].

It is an insoluble, injectable, aluminum-free ready-to-use material and does not require intervention before use. Its radiopacity is 3.84 mm Al [105] and its film thickness is compatible with ISO specification (less than 50 μm). It does not cause any tooth discoloration because of its zirconium oxide ingredients as a radiopacifier [106]. Setting time is four hours (ISO 6876:2001) in normal conditions and working time can be more than four hours at room temperature. The moisture and body temperature lower the setting time. During the root canal obturation, the root canal is not required to be wet. The natural moisture inside the dentinal tubules is enough for setting. On the other hand, overdrying root canal increases setting time up to 10 hours [106]. The flowability of these products increases with the body temperature. Owing to the narrow contact angle, they can easily spread to canal details, irregularities, accessory, and lateral canals [5].

It is osteogenic and biocompatible. It is known that these bioceramics can remain stable in wet conditions and show highly hydrophilic properties [5]. Dentine moisture facilitates the hydration reactions of calcium silicate, thereby, calcium silicate hydrogel and calcium hydroxide are formed [107]. Then, calcium hydroxide combines with calcium phosphate to form hydroxyapatite and water [108]. The water formed reacts again with the calcium silicate; calcium silicate hydrogel, and calcium hydroxide persist. This explains the reason for the high alkaline pH (>12) of the iRoot SP. In addition, its antibacterial activity is attributed to its high pH and active calcium hydroxide diffusion [70]. The formed

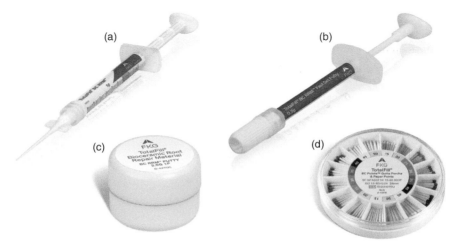

Figure 3.5 TotalFill® examples. *Source:* FKG Dentaire.

hydroxyapatite during setting is shown as the reason to be osteoconductive, and its nanoparticles ensure good adhesion and chemical bonding to dentine [105].

Qu et al. [109] investigated the change of physical properties of pastes at different temperatures under a stereomicroscope. When placed in a temperature increasing environment (25–140 °C) for 10 minutes after mixing, the fluidity of AH Plus increased, while the fluidity of RoekoSeal (Roeko/Coltene/Whaledent, Langenau, Germany) and iRoot SP pastes decreased. It was observed that the porosity of iRoot SP sealer decreased at high temperatures. Moreover, the flow and setting time of RoekoSeal and iRoot SP sealers reduced with the increase of temperature [109].

A study examining the dislocation resistance of iRoot SP and AH Plus observed that both had higher bond strengths than EndoREZ^{TM} and Sealapex (SybronEndo Corporation, Orange, CA) and their values were very close to each other [110]. In addition, another study [111] found no difference between AH Plus and iRoot SP in terms of microleakage, apical sealing, or solubility. AH Plus and iRoot SP sealers were found to provide similar apical sealing [70].

Some studies were also done to evaluate the clinical effect of these sealers regarding postoperative pain, quality of life, and analgesic intake after root canal treatment. Atav Ates et al. [112] compared the AH Plus and iRoot SP sealers in a study conducted on vital teeth filled HEROfill (Micro-Mega Besancon, France) obturation system. They found that there was no significant difference in postoperative pain incidence between groups; only painkiller was taken more in the AH Plus group. Similar to the results of Atav Ates et al. [112], Donmez Ozkan and Aslan [113] found no difference regarding pain and analgesic intake after the obturation with Endoseal MTA, EndoSequence® BC Sealer, and an epoxy resin-based (AH Plus) sealer.

iRoot SP, EndoSequence® BC, and TotalFill® sealers can be used both with or without gutta-percha in root canal obturation [104]. They have their special gutta-perchas (EndoSequence® BC points and TotalFill® BC Points™) (Figure 3.5d) which are impregnated and coated with bioceramic nanoparticles to improve bonding both with sealer and dentine for a gap-free filling. When it is compared with conventional points, BC points are shown not to be cytotoxic [114]. While the standard version of this gutta-percha is manufactured for cold obturation technique, the HiFlow™ version (melts at 150 °C) is for warm bonded obturation techniques. Retreatment procedure is more possible in the presence of gutta-percha [115].

These products are presented in different subtitles to suit the clinician's necessity: HiFlow, injectable paste, putty, and malleable putty. There are similar products of TotalFill®, iRoot, and Endosequence® BC [7]. They are highly biocompatible, bioactive, osteogenic, hydrophilic, and insoluble. They have antibacterial properties thanks to high pH (+12 pH). These products have fast settings and negligible cytotoxicity [116].

3.2.5.2   EndoSequence® BC Sealer HiFlow and TotalFill® BC Sealer HiFlow™

As heat can change the properties of bioceramic sealers, it was a question for clinicians if the warm obturation techniques affect the quality of bioceramic sealers. So, HiFlow formula, which is a sealer that does not change its features with heating, is produced. These products are the variations of their original formulas. Their compositions are not notified by the manufacturers until now [117]. It is a preloaded syringe. It has a lower viscosity and is more radiopaque than the original form. It has a resistance up to 220 °C [7].

3.2.5.3   TotalFill® BC RRM Root Repair Material (RRM)Paste, iRoot BP, EndoSequence® BC Root Repair Material (ERRM) or Bioceramic Root Repair Material (BC RRM) (Brasseler USA, Savannah, GA, USA)

They are ready-to-use and semi-solid premixed bioceramic materials. Their general properties are similar to their original form regarding composition, radiopacity, dimensional stability, insolubility, and physical properties such as the need of water for setting. Their components are calcium silicates, calcium phosphate monobasic, zirconium oxide, tantalum oxide, and thickening agents [115].

Their setting time is two hours and working time is approximately 30 minutes [115]. They were developed for permanent root canal repair (perforations and resorption areas) and surgical applications. They can also be used in pulp capping [115].

3.2.5.4   TotalFill® BC RRM™ Putty, iRoot BP Plus, EndoSequence® BC RRM Putty

They were released as a preloaded jar in the market (Figure 3.5c). They are produced for apexification, retrofilling, and perforation repair treatments. These materials contain zirconium oxide, calcium sulphates, tantalum oxide, calcium silicates, and calcium phosphates [118]. They have higher radiopacity than sealer and RRM materials (approx. 9.17 mm Al) [119]. Total setting time is approximately two hours. Its consistency is slightly thicker and more malleable than TotalFill® BC RRM Paste [115]. In a study by Al-Saudi et al. [120], after pulp capping with TotalFill® BC RRM™ Putty complete dentine bridge formation and an absence of inflammatory pulp response were seen at three weeks and three months after treatment. Also, bridge thickness was higher than NeoMTA Plus (Avalon Biomed Inc., Bradenton, FL, USA) [120].

3.2.5.5   TotalFill® BC RRM™ Fast Set Putty, iRoot FS, EndoSequence® BC RRM Fast Set Puty

The main difference from their original putty form is the short setting time of the material (approximately 20 minutes) (Figure 3.5b) [115]. When these fast set putty materials are used for perforation repair, it is recommended to cover the material with self-cure or dual-cure glass ionomer cement in single-visit treatments [106].

In a study by Jiang et al. [116] it was demonstrated that cell adhesion capacity of fast set putty is more than its original putty form.

3.2.5.6 Well-Root™ ST

Well-Root™ ST (Vericom, Gangwon-Do, Korea) (Figure 3.6c) is a premixed root canal sealer and is supplied in an injectable syringe. Its ingredients are zirconium oxide, calcium silicate, filler, and thickening agents [44, 117]. This is a bioactive permanent obturation material. It is especially produced for permanent root canal treatment and is useful in complicated cases such as perforation, open apex, etc. [5].

Similar to other calcium silicate cements it needs wet conditions to harden. Well-Root™ ST does not shrink during setting and exhibits superior physical properties. The setting time is 25 minutes, but this time may increase up to two-and-a-half hours during root canal treatment [121].

It induces biocompatibility, biomineralization, and osteoconductivity [44, 117]. It shows high angiogenetic properties. It shows chemical bonding to dentine. During and after setting, hydroxyapatite crystals form on its surface. Its pH rises above 12 during the setting. Therefore, it has high antibacterial properties [44, 117]. Olcay et al. [122] found that the angiogenic properties are higher than ProRoot MTA and Biodentine, and biocompatibility is similar to these bioceramics.

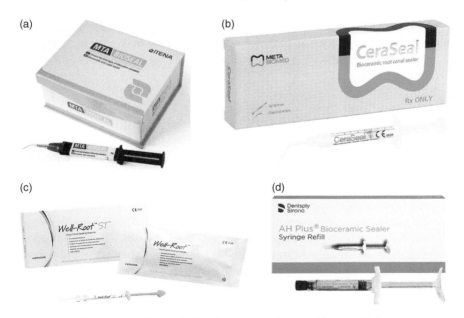

Figure 3.6 Examples for Type 5 hydraulic cements. *Sources:* (a) Itena Clinical. (b) Ceraseal/MetaBiomed. (c). VALDENTAL LTD./https://en.valdental.eu/product/well-root-st-bio-ceramic-root-canal-sealing-material (accessed 9 May 2023). (d) Dentsply Sirona.

3.2.5.7 CeraSeal

CeraSeal (Meta Biomed Co., Cheongju, Korea) (Figure 3.6b) is a premixed root canal sealer that contains calcium silicates, zirconium oxide, and a thickening agent [123].

It has high pH (>12). Its setting time is three-and-a-half hours. It has excellent radiopacity (approximately 8 mm Al). The solubility of this sealer was found more than ISO specification 6876:2012 (3% mass after 24 hours) [124]. It has dimensional stability (neither shrinks, nor expands) [7].

According to the manufacturer [125], it provides superb antimicrobial activity and biocompatibility. Antimicrobial activity and high pH may be attributed to the present calcium hydroxide ($Ca(OH)_2$).

3.2.5.8 MTA Bioseal

MTA Bioseal (Itena, Villepinte, France) (Figure 3.6a) is a bioceramic sealer that contains 13% of MTA. Its formula is based on calcium tungstate, a high-quality radiopacifier that is not linked to discoloration of teeth [126]. It has a double paste component that allows gap-free filling of all root canals including ramifications, lateral canals, and irregularities.

MTA Bioseal is indicated for root canal filling of definitive teeth with gutta-percha points. It is compatible with both cold and thermal condensation techniques (boiling point is over 140 °C) [126]. Its working time is 23 minutes and setting time is two hours. The presence of salicylate resin makes it easy to retreat if needed. MTA Bioseal possesses high values of radiopacity for easy visualization [126].

3.2.5.9 Bio-C Repair

Bio-C Repair (Angelus, Londrina, PR, Brazil) (Figure 3.7d) is a new, calcium silicate-based bioceramic cement. It has been recently placed on the market for reparative or regenerative endodontic treatments with the same applications and the same biological interactions as MTA. But it has improvements in terms of handling and placement [123]. The material's composition includes zirconium oxide as radiopacifier, calcium silicate, calcium oxide, silicon dioxide, iron oxide, calcium aluminate, and dispersing agent [59].

It has favorable biological properties such as inducing cell viability, adhesion and migration, and biomineralization [59, 123]. It has been shown to rapidly stimulate osteoblast differentiation [127]. Based on the results of an in vitro study evaluating the obturation abilities of Bio-C Repair and MTA Repair HP, Bio-C Repair showed perfect obturation ability and low volumetric change [128]. In another study comparing the bonding properties of Biodentine, MTA Repair HP, and Bio-C Repair to dentine, Biodentine was found the most successful, while Bio-C Repair has shown the least bond strength [64].

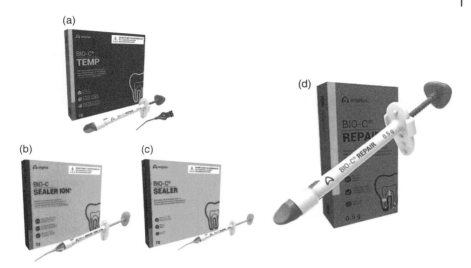

Figure 3.7 Bio-C family. *Sources:* (a) Clinical Research Dental Supplies and Services Inc./https://www.clinicalresearchdental.com/products/angelus-bio-c-temp-bioceramic-intracanal-medication?variant=39404439601206 (accessed 9 May 2023). (b–d) Progressive Healthcare Solutions Pvt Ltd/https://medic-kart.com/shop/angelus-bio-c-sealer/ (accessed 9 May 2023).

3.2.5.10 Bio-C Sealer

Bio-C Sealer (Angelus, Londrina, PR, Brazil) (Figure 3.7c) was launched in 2018 [129]. It is composed of tricalcium silicate, tricalcium aluminate, dicalcium silicate, silicon oxide, calcium oxide, polyethylene glycol, iron oxide, and zirconia oxide [130]. It is also clinically recommended not only as a sealer for root canal obturation [65] but also as a root-end filling material [131].

According to its manufacturer, its radiopacity is 5.5 mm AI [132]. When the Bio-C Sealer's calcium silicate structure comes into contact with local humidity, they hydrate and form a hydrated calcium silicate structure. On the other hand, the formed $Ca(OH)_2$ rapidly decomposes into Ca^{2+} and OH^- ions, thus increasing the pH and preventing bacterial growth in the environment [131]. In addition, Bio-C Sealer has been shown to induce the expression and biomineralization of markers related to bone formation [59] and alkaline phosphatase (ALP) activity [54].

3.2.5.11 Bio-C Temp

Bio-C Temp (Angelus, Londrina, PR, Brazil) (Figure 3.7a) is another calcium silicate-based ready-for-use bioceramic paste for intracanal dressing. It was launched in 2020 [133]. It is marketed in a special syringe. Thanks to the syringe and applicator tips specially produced for the product, the product does not absorb moisture from the environment outside and thus premature hardening is not observed. Its composition consists of the following components: tricalcium silicate, tricalcium aluminate, dicalcium silicate, base resin, calcium oxide, polyethylene glycol, calcium tungstate, and titanium oxide. Tricalcium silicate, dicalcium silicate, and tricalcium aluminate are active components and their function is related to the release of calcium and hydroxyl ions. Base resin is for plasticity, calcium tungstate is for radiopacity, polyethylene glycol is a dispersing agent, and titanium oxide is for pigmentation [134].

According to the manufacturer, it is indicated as an intracanal dressing as an alternative to calcium hydroxide in pulp necrosis, root canal treatment, retreatment cases, external/internal resorptions, perforations, and incomplete rhizogenesis cases. It is recommended to use before using Bio-C Repair, MTA Repair HP, and MTA Angelus. It has also been indicated that it can be also used in pulpotomy, apexification, and endodontic regenerative cases [26].

3.2.5.12 Bio-C Pulpecto

Bio-C Pulpecto (Angelus®, Londrina, PR, Brazil) is the first bioceramic-based material developed to be used during the obturation of root canals in primary teeth. It contains ester glycol salicylate, calcium tungstate, titanium oxide, toluene sulfonamide, silicon dioxide, and calcium silicate [135]. Its pH is 12.7 and its radiopacity is 9 mm Al [135]. Bio-C Pulpecto is biocompatible, can initiate biomineralization and, similar to MTA, it is immunopositive for several osteogenic markers [95]. It has been reported that Bio-C Pulpecto has adequate physicochemical properties, is cytocompatible, and has the potential to induce mineralization [135].

3.2.5.13 Bio-C Sealer ION+

Bio-C Sealer ION+ (Angelus, Londrina, PR, Brazil) (Figure 3.7b) was recently marketed in 2021 as a premixed, ready to use, resin-free and eugenol-free calcium silicate-based bioceramic root canal sealer.

According to the manufacturer, the high flow (23–25 mm) of material helps to reach the accessory channels. Bio-C Sealer ION+ can be used in harmony with single cone, cold and hot gutta-percha techniques. It has <2 μm particle size, ≥7 mm Al radiopacity, ≤240 minutes setting time, ≈12 pH, 21 μm film thickness, 0.5–2.5% solubility and 5–15 MPa resistance to compression [136]. It can set in the presence of moisture in the root canal. In a recent study, it was stated that Bio-C sealer ION+ caused upregulation of CEMP1, CAP and RUNX2 genes, showed successful biocompatibility results, and was a suitable material for clinical use [137].

3.2.5.14 AH Plus Bioceramic Sealer

AH Plus Bioceramic Sealer (Dentsply Sirona, Ballaigues, Switzerland) (Figure 3.6d) has been produced recently. The company claimed that AH Plus Bioceramic Sealer provides an ideal sealing ability. It is biocompatible. It does not contain bismuth oxide. It does not cause discoloration. It is easy to disassemble when retreatment is required. It shows a higher radiopacity than other bioceramic-based sealers. It causes the formation of a very favorable environment for hydroxyapatite formation. It offers low film thickness. It exhibits high wash-out resistance. It can remain stable for a long time in the root canal. It also has lipophilic and hydrophilic properties [138]. There is a need for physicochemical and biological in vitro and in vivo studies for this recently developed product.

3.3 Conclusion

Calcium silicate-based materials are the new future of endodontics. Both the physicochemical and biological properties of bioceramic materials have been improved day by day. There are many alternative products in the market for every endodontic situation and can be used safely thanks to their biocompatible properties.

References

1 Tomaszewska, M.A. (2023). Bond strength of calcium silicate based bioceramic sealers to dentin. Master thesis. Boston University.

2 Šimundić Munitić, M., Poklepović Peričić, T., Utrobičić, A. et al. (2019). Antimicrobial efficacy of commercially available endodontic bioceramic root canal sealers: a systematic review. *PLoS One* 14 (10): e0223575.

3 Al-Haddad, A. and Che Ab Aziz, Z.A. (2016). Bioceramic-based root canal sealers: a review. *International Journal of Biomaterials* 2016: 9753210.

4 Islam, I., Chng, H.K., and Yap, A.U.J. (2006). Comparison of the physical and mechanical properties of MTA and Portland cement. *Journal of Endodontics* 32 (3): 193–197.

5 Bioaggregate Brochure (2022). https://endo.bg/image/data/files/DiaRoot_Booklet.pdf (accessed 28 April 2022).

6 Malhotra, S., Hegde, M.N., and Shetty, C. (2014). Bioceramic technology in endodontics. *British Journal of Medicine and Medical Research* 4 (12): 2446.

7 Camilleri, J. (2021). Current classification of bioceramic materials in endodontics. In: *Bioceramic Materials in Clinical Endodontics* (ed. S. Drukteinis and J. Camilleri), 1–87. Springer.

8 de Freitas Lima, S.M., Rezende, T.M.B., Silva, P.A.O. et al. (2020). Improvement of reparative bioceramics in endodontics – a critical review. *Biomedical Journal of Scientific & Technical Research* 24 (3): 18306–18310.

9 Shen, Y., Peng, B., Yang, Y. et al. (2015). What do different tests tell about the mechanical and biological properties of bioceramic materials? *Endodontic Topics* 32 (1): 47–85.

10 Tawil, P.Z., Duggan, D.J., and Galicia, J.C. (2015). Mineral trioxide aggregate (MTA): its history, composition, and clinical applications. *Compendium of Continuing Education in Dentistry (Jamesburg, NJ: 1995)* 36 (4): 247–252. quiz 54, 64.

11 Song, W., Sun, W., Chen, L., and Yuan, Z. (2020). In vivo biocompatibility and bioactivity of calcium silicate-based bioceramics in endodontics. *Frontiers in Bioengineering and Biotechnology* 8: 580954.

12 Kim, D.-H., Jang, J.-H., Lee, B.-N. et al. (2018). Anti-inflammatory and mineralization effects of proroot MTA and endocem MTA in studies of human and rat dental pulps in vitro and in vivo. *Journal of Endodontics* 44 (10): 1534–1541.

13 Ber, B.S., Hatton, J.F., and Stewart, G.P. (2007). Chemical modification of ProRoot MTA to improve handling characteristics and decrease setting time. *Journal of Endodontics* 33 (10): 1231–1234.

14 Camilleri, J. (2008). The chemical composition of mineral trioxide aggregate. *Journal of Conservative Dentistry: JCD* 11 (4): 141.

15 Rao, A., Rao, A., and Shenoy, R. (2009). Mineral trioxide aggregate – a review. *Journal of Clinical Pediatric Dentistry* 34 (1): 1–8.

16 Salehimehr, G., Nobahar, S., Hosseini-Zijoud, S.-M., and Yari, S. (2014). Comparison of physical & chemical properties of Angelus MTA and new endodontic restorative material. *Journal of Applied Pharmaceutical Science* 4 (7): 105–109.

17 Camilleri, J. and Gandolfi, M. (2010). Evaluation of the radiopacity of calcium silicate cements containing different radiopacifiers. *International Endodontic Journal* 43 (1): 21–30.

18 Sisli, S.N. and Ozbas, H. (2017). Comparative micro–computed tomographic evaluation of the sealing quality of ProRoot MTA and MTA Angelus apical plugs placed with various techniques. *Journal of Endodontics* 43 (1): 147–151.

19 Camilleri, J., Sorrentino, F., and Damidot, D. (2013). Investigation of the hydration and bioactivity of radiopacified tricalcium silicate cement, Biodentine and MTA Angelus. *Dental Materials* 29 (5): 580–593.

20 Malhotra, N., Agarwal, A., and Mala, K. (2013). Mineral trioxide aggregate: a review of physical properties. *Compendium of Continuing Education in Dentistry (Jamesburg, NJ: 1995)* 34 (2): e25–e32.

21 Gandolfi, M., Siboni, F., and Prati, C. (2012). Chemical–physical properties of TheraCal, a novel light-curable MTA-like material for pulp capping. *International Endodontic Journal* 45 (6): 571–579.

22 Cintra, L.T.A., Benetti, F., de Azevedo Queiroz, Í.O. et al. (2017). Cytotoxicity, biocompatibility, and biomineralization of the new high-plasticity MTA material. *Journal of Endodontics* 43 (5): 774–778.

23 Gandolfi, M.G., Siboni, F., Botero, T. et al. (2015). Calcium silicate and calcium hydroxide materials for pulp capping: biointeractivity, porosity, solubility and bioactivity of current formulations. *Journal of Applied Biomaterials & Functional Materials* 13 (1): 43–60.

24 De-Deus, G., Audi, C., Murad, C. et al. (2008). Similar expression of through-and-through fluid movement along orthograde apical plugs of MTA Bio™ and white Portland cement. *International Endodontic Journal* 41 (12): 1047–1053.

25 Borges, A.H., Guedes, O.A., Volpato, L.E.R. et al. (2017). Physicochemical properties of MTA and Portland cement after addition of Aloe vera. *Iranian Endodontic Journal* 12 (3): 312.

26 Guerreiro, J., Ochoa-Rodrígez, V., Rodrigues, E. et al. (2021). Antibacterial activity, cytocompatibility and effect of Bio-C Temp bioceramic intracanal medicament on osteoblast biology. *International Endodontic Journal* 54 (7): 1155–1165.

27 MTA BIO Brochure (2022). https://www.cerkamed.com/product/bio-mta-plus/ (accessed 21 July 2022).

28 Lessa, F.C.R., Aranha, A.M.F., Hebling, J., and Costa, C.A.S. (2010). Cytotoxic effects of White-MTA and MTA-Bio cements on odontoblast-like cells (MDPC-23). *Brazilian Dental Journal* 21: 24–31.

29 Talabani, R.M., Garib, B.T., and Masaeli, R. (2020). Bioactivity and physicochemical properties of three calcium silicate-based cements: an in vitro study. *BioMed Research International* 2020: 9582165.

30 Sogukpinar, A. and Arikan, V. (2020). Comparative evaluation of four endodontic biomaterials and calcium hydroxide regarding their effect on fracture resistance of simulated immature teeth. *European Journal of Paediatric Dentistry* 21 (1): 23–28.

31 Tanalp, J., Karapınar-Kazandağ, M., Dölekoğlu, S., and Kayahan, M.B. (2013). Comparison of the radiopacities of different root-end filling and repair materials. *The Scientific World Journal* 2013: 594950.

32 MM MTA Brochure (2022). MM-MTA™ state-of-the-art endodontic repair cement. https://micro-mega.com/wp-content/uploads/2018/03/MM-MTA_brochure-1.pdf (accessed 21 July 2022).

33 Khalil, I., Naaman, A., and Camilleri, J. (2015). Investigation of a novel mechanically mixed mineral trioxide aggregate (MM-MTA™). *International Endodontic Journal* 48 (8): 757–767.

34 Kum, K., Kim, E.C., Yoo, Y.J. et al. (2014). Trace metal contents of three tricalcium silicate materials: MTA Angelus, Micro Mega MTA and Bioaggregate. *International Endodontic Journal* 47 (7): 704–710.

35 Onay, E.O., Yurtcu, E., Terzi, Y.K. et al. (2018). Odontogenic effects of two calcium silicate-based biomaterials in human dental pulp cells. *Advances in Clinical and Experimental Medicine* 27 (11): 1541–1547.

36 Margunato, S., Taşlı, P.N., Aydın, S. et al. (2015). In vitro evaluation of ProRoot MTA, Biodentine, and MM-MTA on human alveolar bone marrow stem cells in terms of biocompatibility and mineralization. *Journal of Endodontics* 41 (10): 1646–1652.

37 Kim, S., Kim, S., Park, J.-W. et al. (2017). Comparison of the percentage of voids in the canal filling of a calcium silicate-based sealer and gutta percha cones using two obturation techniques. *Materials* 10 (10): 1170.

38 Kim, S.R., Kwak, S.W., Lee, J.-K. et al. (2019). Efficacy and retrievability of root canal filling using calcium silicate-based and epoxy resin-based root canal sealers with matched obturation techniques. *Australian Endodontic Journal* 45 (3): 337–345.

39 Torabinejad, M., Parirokh, M., and Dummer, P.M. (2018). Mineral trioxide aggregate and other bioactive endodontic cements: an updated overview – part II: other clinical applications and complications. *International Endodontic Journal* 51 (3): 284–317.

40 EndoSeal MTA Brochure. https://maruchiusa.com/pages/endoseal-mta (accessed 21 July 2022).

41 Lim, E.-S., Park, Y.-B., Kwon, Y.-S. et al. (2015). Physical properties and biocompatibility of an injectable calcium-silicate-based root canal sealer: in vitro and in vivo study. *BMC Oral Health* 15 (1): 1–7.

42 Jafari, F. and Jafari, S. (2017). Composition and physicochemical properties of calcium silicate based sealers: a review article. *Journal of Clinical and Experimental Dentistry* 9 (10): e1249.

43 Seo, D.-G., Lee, D., Kim, Y.-M. et al. (2019). Biocompatibility and mineralization activity of three calcium silicate-based root canal sealers compared to conventional resin-based sealer in human dental pulp stem cells. *Materials* 12 (15): 2482.

44 Lee, J.K., Kim, S., Lee, S. et al. (2019). In vitro comparison of biocompatibility of calcium silicate-based root canal sealers. *Materials* 12 (15): 2411.

45 Upadhyay, S.T., Purayil, T.P., and Ginjupalli, K. (2017). Comparative evaluation of fracture resistance of endodontically treated teeth obturated with pozzolan-based MTA sealer and epoxy resin-based sealer: an in vitro study. *World Journal of Dentistry* 8 (1): 37–40.

46 Lee, D.-S., Lim, M.-J., Choi, Y. et al. (2016). Tooth discoloration induced by a novel mineral trioxide aggregate-based root canal sealer. *European Journal of Dentistry* 10 (03): 403–407.

47 Hwang, J.H., Chung, J., Na, H.S. et al. (2015). Comparison of bacterial leakage resistance of various root canal filling materials and methods: confocal laser-scanning microscope study. *Scanning* 37 (6): 422–428.

48 Mak, S.T., Leong, X.F., Tew, I.M. et al. (2022). In vitro evaluation of the antibacterial activity of EndoSeal MTA, iRoot SP, and AH Plus against planktonic bacteria. *Materials* 15 (6): 2012.

49 Dastorani, M., Shourvarzi, B., Nojoumi, F., and Ajami, M. (2021). Comparison of bacterial microleakage of endoseal MTA sealer and pro-root MTA in root perforation. *Journal of Dentistry* 22 (2): 96.

50 Forghani, M., Gharechahi, M., and Karimpour, S. (2016). In vitro evaluation of tooth discoloration induced by MTA Fillapex and iRoot SP endodontic sealers. *International Congress of Iranian Association of Endodontists*. SID.

51 Sönmez, I., Oba, A., Sönmez, D., and Almaz, M. (2012). In vitro evaluation of apical microleakage of a new MTA-based sealer. *European Archives of Paediatric Dentistry* 13 (5): 252–255.

52 MTA Angelus Brochure (2022). MTA fillapex endodontic sealer. https://www. angelusdental.com/img/arquivos/mta_fillapex_technical_profile_download.pdf (accessed 21 July 2022).

53 Viapiana, R., Flumignan, D., Guerreiro-Tanomaru, J. et al. (2014). Physicochemical and mechanical properties of zirconium oxide and niobium oxide modified Portland cement-based experimental endodontic sealers. *International Endodontic Journal* 47 (5): 437–448.

54 Pedrosa, M.S., Alves, T., Nogueira, F.N. et al. (2021). Cytotoxicity and cytokine production by calcium silicate-based materials on periodontal ligament stem cells. *Brazilian Dental Journal* 32: 65–74.

55 Zmener, O., Lalis, R.M., Pameijer, C.H. et al. (2012). Reaction of rat subcutaneous connective tissue to a mineral trioxide aggregate–based and a zinc oxide and eugenol sealer. *Journal of Endodontics* 38 (9): 1233–1238.

56 Gomes-Filho, J.E., Watanabe, S., Cintra, L.T.A. et al. (2013). Effect of MTA-based sealer on the healing of periapical lesions. *Journal of Applied Oral Science* 21: 235–242.

57 Silva, E.J.N.L., Carvalho, N.K., Prado, M.C. et al. (2016). Push-out bond strength of injectable pozzolan-based root canal sealer. *Journal of Endodontics* 42 (11): 1656–1659.

58 Zhou, H.-m., Du, T.-f., Shen, Y. et al. (2015). In vitro cytotoxicity of calcium silicate–containing endodontic sealers. *Journal of Endodontics* 41 (1): 56–61.

59 Benetti, F., Queiroz, Í.O.A., Cosme-Silva, L. et al. (2019). Cytotoxicity, biocompatibility and biomineralization of a new ready-for-use bioceramic repair material. *Brazilian Dental Journal* 30: 325–332.

60 Beegum, M.F., George, S., Anandaraj, S. et al. (2021). Comparative evaluation of diffused calcium and hydroxyl ion release from three different Indirect pulp capping agents in permanent teeth – an in vitro study. *The Saudi Dental Journal* 33 (8): 1149–1153.

61 Hardan, L., Mancino, D., Bourgi, R. et al. (2022). Bond strength of adhesive systems to calcium silicate-based materials: a systematic review and meta-analysis of in vitro studies. *Gels* 8 (5): 311.

62 TheraCal LC Brochure (2022). https://www.bisco.com/assets/1/22/TheraCal_LC_Brochure3.pdf (accessed 22 July 2022).

63 TheraCal PT Brochure (2022). https://nudent.co.th/product/theracal-pt/ (accessed 21 July 2022).

64 Rodríguez-Lozano, F.J., López-García, S., Garcia-Bernal, D. et al. (2021). Cytocompatibility and bioactive properties of the new dual-curing resin-modified calcium silicate-based material for vital pulp therapy. *Clinical Oral Investigations* 25 (8): 5009–5024.

65 Sanz, J.L., Soler-Doria, A., López-García, S. et al. (2021). Comparative biological properties and mineralization potential of 3 endodontic materials for vital pulp therapy: Theracal PT, Theracal LC, and biodentine on human dental pulp stem cells. *Journal of Endodontics* 47 (12): 1896–1906.

66 Elbanna, A., Atta, D., and Sherief, D.I. (2022). In vitro bioactivity of newly introduced dual-cured resin-modified calcium silicate cement. *Dental Research Journal* 19: 1–11.

67 Zhu, L., Yang, J., Zhang, J., and Peng, B. (2014). A comparative study of BioAggregate and ProRoot MTA on adhesion, migration, and attachment of human dental pulp cells. *Journal of Endodontics* 40 (8): 1118–1123.

68 Lu D and Zhou S. (2009). High strength biological cement composition and using the same. Google Patents US7553362B2, filed 26 October 2006 and issued 30 June 2009

69 Camilleri, J., Sorrentino, F., and Damidot, D. (2015). Characterization of un-hydrated and hydrated BioAggregate™ and MTA Angelus™. *Clinical Oral Investigations* 19 (3): 689–698.

70 Zhang, H., Pappen, F.G., and Haapasalo, M. (2009). Dentin enhances the antibacterial effect of mineral trioxide aggregate and bioaggregate. *Journal of Endodontics* 35 (2): 221–224.

71 Koch, K., Brave, D., and Nasseh, A.A. (2012). A review of bioceramic technology in endodontics. *CE Article* 4: 6–12.

72 Kossev, A.D. and Stefanov, V. (2009). Ceramics-based sealersas new alternative to currently used endodontic sealers. *Roots* 1: 42–48.

73 Yuan, Z., Peng, B., Jiang, H. et al. (2010). Effect of bioaggregate on mineral-associated gene expression in osteoblast cells. *Journal of Endodontics* 36 (7): 1145–1148.

74 Jung, J.Y., Woo, S.M., Lee, B.N. et al. (2015). Effect of Biodentine and Bioaggregate on odontoblastic differentiation via mitogen-activated protein kinase pathway in human dental pulp cells. *International Endodontic Journal* 48 (2): 177–184.

75 Hashem, A.A.R. and Amin, S.A.W. (2012). The effect of acidity on dislodgment resistance of mineral trioxide aggregate and bioaggregate in furcation perforations: an in vitro comparative study. *Journal of Endodontics* 38 (2): 245–249.

76 Amin, S.A.W. and Gawdat, S.I. (2018). Retention of BioAggregate and MTA as coronal plugs after intracanal medication for regenerative endodontic procedures: an ex vivo study. *Restorative Dentistry & Endodontics.* 43 (3): e18.

77 Biodentine Brochure (2022). https://www.septodontcorp.com/technology-and-products/endodontics-and-restorative/biodentine/ (accessed 6 July 2023).

78 Lipski, M., Nowicka, A., Kot, K. et al. (2018). Factors affecting the outcomes of direct pulp capping using Biodentine. *Clinical Oral Investigations* 22 (5): 2021–2029.

79 About, I. (2018). Recent trends in tricalcium silicates for vital pulp therapy. *Current Oral Health Reports* 5: 178–185.

80 Grech, L., Mallia, B., and Camilleri, J. (2013). Investigation of the physical properties of tricalcium silicate cement-based root-end filling materials. *Dental Materials* 29 (2): e20–e28.

81 Lai, Y., Yang, M.-L., and Lee, S.-Y. (2003). Microhardness and color changes of human dentin with repeated intracoronal bleaching. *Operative Dentistry* 28 (6): 786–792.

82 Malkondu, Ö., Kazandağ, M.K., and Kazazoğlu, E. (2014). A review on biodentine, a contemporary dentine replacement and repair material. *BioMed Research International* 2014: 160951.

83 Luo, Z., Li, D., Kohli, M.R. et al. (2014). Effect of Biodentine™ on the proliferation, migration and adhesion of human dental pulp stem cells. *Journal of Dentistry* 42 (4): 490–497.

84 Nowicka, A., Lipski, M., Parafiniuk, M. et al. (2013). Response of human dental pulp capped with biodentine and mineral trioxide aggregate. *Journal of Endodontics* 39 (6): 743–747.

85 Vouzara, T., Dimosiari, G., Koulaouzidou, E.A., and Economides, N. (2018). Cytotoxicity of a new calcium silicate endodontic sealer. *Journal of Endodontics* 44 (5): 849–852.

86 Siboni, F., Taddei, P., Zamparini, F. et al. (2017). Properties of BioRoot RCS, a tricalcium silicate endodontic sealer modified with povidone and polycarboxylate. *International Endodontic Journal* 50: e120–e136.

87 Septodont BioRoot RCS Brochure (2022). A bioactive breakthroug. https://cdn2.hubspot.net/hubfs/4299081/Endo%20resto/BioRoot-US.pdf?utm_campaign=US%20Campaign&utm_medium=email&_hsmi=82854862&_hsenc=p2ANqtz-_CFMa3H9gedDfm36cUgDiK06VA4I-WDw6Ce9LPigJo7IEv2CyndmLrFtiAroe2fqig MKGaNIzt0zLUmP8pX9-vbA3-UnEDDytZPaokImnkwybFYQ8&utm_content=82854862&utm_source=hs_automation (accesed 22 April 2022).

88 Donnermeyer, D., Vahdat-Pajouh, N., Schäfer, E., and Dammaschke, T. (2019). Influence of the final irrigation solution on the push-out bond strength of calcium silicate-based, epoxy resin-based and silicone-based endodontic sealers. *Odontology* 107 (2): 231–236.

89 Arias-Moliz, M. and Camilleri, J. (2016). The effect of the final irrigant on the antimicrobial activity of root canal sealers. *Journal of Dentistry* 52: 30–36.

90 Matsumoto, S., Hayashi, M., Suzuki, Y. et al. (2013). Calcium ions released from mineral trioxide aggregate convert the differentiation pathway of C2C12 cells into osteoblast lineage. *Journal of Endodontics* 39 (1): 68–75.

91 Jeanneau, C., Giraud, T., Laurent, P., and About, I. (2019). BioRoot RCS extracts modulate the early mechanisms of periodontal inflammation and regeneration. *Journal of Endodontics* 45 (8): 1016–1023.

92 Alsubait, S., Albader, S., Alajlan, N. et al. (2019). Comparison of the antibacterial activity of calcium silicate-and epoxy resin-based endodontic sealers against Enterococcus faecalis biofilms: a confocal laser-scanning microscopy analysis. *Odontology* 107 (4): 513–520.

93 MTA BioSeal product content (2022). https://itena-clinical.com/en/ endodontics/24-mta-biorep.html (accesed 23 July 2022).

94 MTA BioSeal brochure (2022). https://itena-clinical.com/en/index. php?controller=attachment&id_attachment=557. (accesed 23 July 2022).

95 Cosme-Silva, L., Gomes-Filho, J., Benetti, F. et al. (2019). Biocompatibility and immunohistochemical evaluation of a new calcium silicate-based cement, Bio-C Pulpo. *International Endodontic Journal* 52 (5): 689–700.

96 Pelepenko, L.E., Saavedra, F., Antunes, T.B.M. et al. (2021). Investigation of a modified hydraulic calcium silicate-based material – Bio-C Pulpo. *Brazilian Oral Research* 35: e077.

97 Delfino, M.M., de Abreu Jampani, J.L., Lopes, C.S. et al. (2021). Comparison of Bio-C Pulpo and MTA Repair HP with White MTA: effect on liver parameters and evaluation of biocompatibility and bioactivity in rats. *International Endodontic Journal* 54 (9): 1597–1613.

98 MTA Repair HP Brochure (2022). Bioceramic hugh-plasticity reparative cement. https://angelus.ind.br/assets/uploads/2020/09/Folder-MTA-Repair-HP-ING-USA-Digital.pdf (accessed 21 July 2022).

99 Palczewska-Komsa, M., Kaczor-Wiankowska, K., and Nowicka, A. (2021). New bioactive calcium silicate cement mineral trioxide aggregate repair high plasticity (MTA HP) – a systematic review. *Materials* 14 (16): 4573.

100 Ferreira, C., Sassone, L.M., Gonçalves, A.S. et al. (2019). Physicochemical, cytotoxicity and in vivo biocompatibility of a high-plasticity calcium-silicate based material. *Scientific Reports* 9 (1): 1–11.

101 Marciano, M.A., Costa, R.M., Camilleri, J. et al. (2014). Assessment of color stability of white mineral trioxide aggregate angelus and bismuth oxide in contact with tooth structure. *Journal of Endodontics* 40 (8): 1235–1240.

102 Tanomaru-Filho, M., Morales, V., da Silva, G.F. et al. (2012). Compressive strength and setting time of MTA and Portland cement associated with different radiopacifying agents. *International Scholarly Research Notices* 2012: 1–4.

103 Amoroso-Silva, P.A., Marciano, M.A., Guimaraes, B.M. et al. (2014). Apical adaptation, sealing ability and push-out bond strength of five root-end filling materials. *Brazilian Oral Research* 28: 1–6.

104 Fernández, R., Restrepo, J., Aristizábal, D., and Álvarez, L. (2016). Evaluation of the filling ability of artificial lateral canals using calcium silicate-based and epoxy resin-based endodontic sealers and two gutta-percha filling techniques. *International Endodontic Journal* 49 (4): 365–373.

105 Tyagi, S., Mishra, P., and Tyagi, P. (2013). Evolution of root canal sealers: an insight story. *European Journal of General Dentistry* 2 (03): 199–218.

106 Chang, J.W.W., Praisarnti, C., and Neelakantan, P. (2017). Increasing use of bioceramics in endodontics: a narrative review. *Oral Health Group* 2017 https:// www.oralhealthgroup.com/features/increasing-use-of-bioceramics-in-endodontics-a-narrative-review.

107 Richardson, I.G. (2008). The calcium silicate hydrates. *Cement and Concrete Research* 38 (2): 137–158.

108 Yang, Q., Troczynski, T., and Liu, D.-M. (2002). Influence of apatite seeds on the synthesis of calcium phosphate cement. *Biomaterials* 23 (13): 2751–2760.

109 Qu, W., Bai, W., Liang, Y.-H., and Gao, X.-J. (2016). Influence of warm vertical compaction technique on physical properties of root canal sealers. *Journal of Endodontics* 42 (12): 1829–1833.

110 Ersahan, S. and Aydin, C. (2010). Dislocation resistance of iRoot SP, a calcium silicate–based sealer, from radicular dentine. *Journal of Endodontics* 36 (12): 2000–2002.

111 Ersahan, S. and Aydin, C. (2013). Solubility and apical sealing characteristics of a new calcium silicate-based root canal sealer in comparison to calcium hydroxide-, methacrylate resin-and epoxy resin-based sealers. *Acta Odontologica Scandinavica* 71 (3–4): 857–862.

112 Atav Ates, A., Dumani, A., Yoldas, O., and Unal, I. (2019). Post-obturation pain following the use of carrier-based system with AH Plus or iRoot SP sealers: a randomized controlled clinical trial. *Clinical Oral Investigations* 23 (7): 3053–3061.

113 Aslan, T. and Dönmez Özkan, H. (2021). The effect of two calcium silicate-based and one epoxy resin-based root canal sealer on postoperative pain: a randomized controlled trial. *International Endodontic Journal* 54 (2): 190–197.

114 Meneses, C.B., Gambini, A.F., Olivi, L.T. et al. (2019). Effect of CPoint, EndoSequence BC, and gutta-percha points on viability and gene expression of periodontal ligament fibroblasts. *European Endodontic Journal* 4 (2): 57.

115 FKG Broshure (2022). Endodontics. https://www.fkg.ch/endodontics (accessed 23 July 2022).

116 Jiang, Y., Zheng, Q., Zhou, X. et al. (2014). A comparative study on root canal repair materials: a cytocompatibility assessment in L929 and MG63 cells. *The Scientific World Journal* 2014: 463826.

117 Donnermeyer, D., Bürklein, S., Dammaschke, T., and Schäfer, E. (2019). Endodontic sealers based on calcium silicates: a systematic review. *Odontology* 107 (4): 421–436.

118 Chu, J.H., Chia, K.Y., Qui, A.L. et al. (2020). The effects of sodium hypochlorite and ethylenediaminetetraacetic acid on the microhardness of Mineral Trioxide Aggregate and TotalFill Bioceramic Putty. *Australian Endodontic Journal* 46 (1): 33–39.

119 Zamparini, F., Siboni, F., Prati, C. et al. (2019). Properties of calcium silicate-monobasic calcium phosphate materials for endodontics containing tantalum pentoxide and zirconium oxide. *Clinical Oral Investigations* 23 (1): 445–457.

120 Al-Saudi, K.W., Nabih, S.M., Farghaly, A.M., and Abo Hager, E.A.-A. (2019). Pulpal repair after direct pulp capping with new bioceramic materials: a comparative histological study. *The Saudi Dental Journal* 31 (4): 469–475.

121 Reszka, P., Nowicka, A., Lipski, M. et al. (2016). A comparative chemical study of calcium silicate-containing and epoxy resin-based root canal sealers. *BioMed Research International* 2016: 1–8.

122 Olcay, K., Taşli, P.N., Güven, E.P. et al. (2020). Effect of a novel bioceramic root canal sealer on the angiogenesis-enhancing potential of assorted human odontogenic stem cells compared with principal tricalcium silicate-based cements. *Journal of Applied Oral Science* 28: e20190215.

123 López-García, S., Myong-Hyun, B., Lozano, A. et al. (2020). Cytocompatibility, bioactivity potential, and ion release of three premixed calcium silicate-based sealers. *Clinical Oral Investigations* 24 (5): 1749–1759.

124 Kharouf, N., Arntz, Y., Eid, A. et al. (2020). Physicochemical and antibacterial properties of novel, premixed calcium silicate-based sealer compared to powder–liquid bioceramic sealer. *Journal of Clinical Medicine* 9 (10): 3096.

125 META BIOMED Brochure. https://www.meta-biomed.com/ (accesed 23 July).

126 ITENA Brochure. (2022). https://itena-clinical.com/en/endodontics/53-mta-bioseal.html (accesed 23 July 2022).

127 Santiago, M.C., Gomes-Cornélio, A.L., de Oliveira, L.A. et al. (2021). Calcium silicate-based cements cause environmental stiffness and show diverse potential to induce osteogenesis in human osteoblastic cells. *Scientific Reports* 11 (1): 1–11.

128 Torres, F.F.E., Pinto, J.C., Figueira, G.O. et al. (2021). A micro-computed tomographic study using a novel test model to assess the filling ability and volumetric changes of bioceramic root repair materials. *Restorative Dentistry & Endodontics* 46 (1): 1–8.

129 Zordan-Bronzel, C.L., Torres, F.F.E., Tanomaru-Filho, M. et al. (2019). Evaluation of physicochemical properties of a new calcium silicate–based sealer, Bio-C Sealer. *Journal of Endodontics* 45 (10): 1248–1252.

130 Silva, E.C.A., Tanomaru-Filho, M., da Silva, G.F. et al. (2020). Biocompatibility and bioactive potential of new calcium silicate–based endodontic sealers: Bio-C Sealer and Sealer Plus BC. *Journal of Endodontics* 46 (10): 1470–1477.

131 Okamura, T., Chen, L., Tsumano, N. et al. (2020). Biocompatibility of a high-plasticity, calcium silicate-based, ready-to-use material. *Materials* 13 (21): 4770.

132 Bio-C Sealer Brochure (2022). Bioceramic root canal sealer ready to use. https://angelus.ind.br/assets/uploads/2019/12/BIO-C®-SEALER-Technical-Scientific-Profile-ENGLISH.pdf (accessed 21 July 2022).

133 Villa, N., Santos, V.V.D., Costa, U.M. et al. (2020). A new calcium silicate-based root canal dressing: physical and chemical properties, cytotoxicity and dentinal tubule penetration. *Brazilian Dental Journal* 31: 598–604.

134 Bio-C Temp Brochure. (2022). Bio-C temp. https://www.angelusdental.com/products/details/id/214 (accessed 22 July 2022).

135 Ochoa Rodriguez, V.M., Tanomaru-Filho, M., Rodrigues, E.M. et al. (2021). Physicochemical properties and effect of bioceramic root canal filling for primary teeth on osteoblast biology. *Journal of Applied Oral Science* 29: e20200870.

136 Bio-C Sealer ION+ Brochure. (2022). https://www.angelusdental.com/img/arquivos/bio_c_sealer_ion_angelus_dental.pdf (accessed 21 July 2022).

137 Sanz, J., López-García, S., Lozano, A. et al. (2021). Microstructural composition, ion release, and bioactive potential of new premixed calcium silicate–based endodontic sealers indicated for warm vertical compaction technique. *Clinical Oral Investigations* 25 (3): 1451–1462.

138 AH Plus Bioceramic Sealer Brochure. (2022). AH Plus bioceramic sealer. https://www.dentsplysirona.com/en-us/discover/discover-by-brand/ah-plus-bioceramic-sealer.html (accessed 21 July 2022).

4

Bioceramics: Root-End Filling Material

Sanjay Miglani[1], Swadheena Patro[2], Ankita Mohanty[3], and Antarikshya Das[4]

[1] Department of Conservative Dentistry & Endodontics, Faculty of Dentistry, Jamia Millia Islamia (A Central University), New Delhi, India

[2] Department of Conservative and Endodontics, Kalinga Institute of Dental Sciences, Kiit University (deemed to be), Odisha, India

[3] Conservative Dentistry and Endodontics Anew Cosmetics Centre, Bangalore, Karnataka, India

[4] Department of Conservative Dentistry and Endodontics, Kalinga Institute of Dental Sciences, Kiit University (deemed to be), Odisha, India

CONTENTS

Bioceramics in Endodontics, First Edition. Edited by Viresh Chopra.
© 2024 John Wiley & Sons, Inc. Published 2024 by John Wiley & Sons, Inc.
Companion website: www.wiley.com/go/chopra/bioceramicsinendodontics

4.1 Introduction

The primary goal of an endodontic treatment remains the chemomechanical disinfection of the root canal system, thereby leading to the removal of necrotic tissue and a decrease in bacterial load [1]. Although conventional treatment protocol must be considered first, considering it is more conservative, occasionally, the surgical approach proves to be inevitable [2]. Endodontic surgery typically entails resection of the apical portion of the root, followed by root-end canal preparation and filling. The purpose of the retrograde filling is to create an apical seal around the canal, prohibiting microbes and related toxins from escaping into the periradicular tissues [3]. Therefore, it is safe to state that the objective of performing an endodontic surgery is to hermetically seal the root canal system and facilitate regeneration by eradicating bacterial contamination [4].

Endodontic materials in clinical use often have to meet certain requirements. They should be biocompatible, bioactive, should possess antimicrobial activity, be visible in radiographs, nonstaining to the tooth structures, dimensionally stable, should be easy to replace yet provide the best quality seal with hard tissues, and should have optimum mechanical strength [5–11]. It is evident that no material used in clinical dentistry, including endodontics, conforms with all the above-mentioned criteria.

In the mid-1990s, mineral trioxide aggregate (MTA) was the introductory bioceramic material which, on its clinical use for root-end filling, aided in the development of numerous other hybrid or bioceramic materials. Essentially all bioceramic materials are biocompatible; they do differ in certain mechanical properties such as setting time, compressive strengths, etc. In conjunction to be used as retrograde fillings, these materials are utilized for pulp capping, repairing perforations, treatment of teeth with open apexes, and correction of defects caused by resorption. They are also employed as orthograde (apical) root fillings. Except for MTA, there isn't much available literature on bioceramic materials, although it is expanding quickly.

This chapter emphasizes the properties, performance, application, and drawbacks of different bioceramics in endodontics when used in periradicular surgery as root-end filling materials [12].

4.2 Microsurgical Endodontics

As quoted, *Endodontic surgery is defined as a surgical procedure on exceptionally small and complex structures with an operating microscope.* Modern techniques use ultrasonic devices that cut with almost negligent or no bevel, producing significantly better clinical results in contrast with carbide round burs that give a bevel of 45° when used for root-end resection. The goal of a steep bevel is to facilitate more visibility of the root end during the procedure; however, this often leads to more damage leading to a large osteotomy.

In contemporary techniques, along with using ultrasonic devices, microscopes aid in performing the surgery with precision thereby providing a more predictable outcome of the procedure [13].

4.3 History

According to Saxena et al. almost every dental restorative material currently in use has been recommended to be used for root-end filling [14]; among them are amalgam, glass ionomer cement, gold foil, super ethoxy-benzoic acid (SuperEBA), gutta-percha, and intermediate restorative material (IRM).

Farrar (1884), followed by Rhein (1897), placed amalgam as a root-end filling material [15]. Abundant research supported the usage of amalgam for retrograde filling because of high success rates. However, it had its share of disadvantages such as corrosion, leakage, moisture sensitivity, tin and mercury contamination, preparation of retrograde cavities that require undercuts, etc.; therefore, amalgam is no more considered as the material of choice [16–18].

Schuster in 1913 introduced gold foil for root-end filling; however, as a result of the complexities involving the placement, finishing, and high cost, it could not be used routinely [15].

In literature, there has been very little discussion about the utilization of GP as a root-end filling material because it causes microleakage, owing to the porous nature of the material. However, Amagasa et al. in 1989 reported a good success rate with gutta-percha being used for root-end filling [19].

Zinc oxide eugenol (ZOE), an otherwise weak cement because of poor mechanical properties and high solubility, was modified to IRM and SuperEBA to revamp its mechanical properties. For its good sealing ability, Hendra in 1970 proposed SuperEBA as a root-end filling material [20]. In a similar vein, a study conducted by Bondra et al. in 1989 concluded that IRM could be used as retrograde filling because it had remarkably less leakage as compared to amalgam. However, tissue irritation, difficult handling properties, sensitivity to moisture, and solubility are all characteristics that could not be ignored [21].

A composite resin developed by Bowen, stated to be hydrophobic in nature, limits its bonding to dentin (a wet substrate); therefore, a dry field and dentin bonding agents become indispensable for a composite to bond. Moisture control of the targeted area is required to allow predictable sealing and, as moisture is very often evident during the placement of a root-end filling, the use of composite resin in periapical surgery for the root-end filling was perhaps limited [13].

Among the major developments in reparative dentistry was the emergence of bioceramics as a new group of restorative materials in the early 1990s. Koch and Brave defined bioceramics as "ceramic products or components employed in medical and dental applications, mainly as implants and replacements that have osteoinductive properties." [22]

Numerous authors have published studies comparing the characteristics of MTA as a retrograde material to those of other materials since 1993. The time frame required for *Staphylococcus epidermidis* to infiltrate a 3-mm layer of retrograde fill made of amalgam, SuperEBA, IRM, or MTA was assessed in one study. Majorly, all samples containing amalgam, SuperEBA, or IRM showed leakage between 6 and 57 days, whereas the majority of samples containing MTA exhibited negligible leakage during the 90-day study period [23].

Many such studies backed MTA as a root-end filling material. Therefore, MTA along with other bioceramic cement will be discussed in detail in this chapter.

4.4 Properties of Root-End Filling Material

The primary goal of root-end filling material placement following root resection and root-end preparation is to hermetically secure the root canal system, which will restrict either the microorganisms or their by-products from leaving or entering the canal which may result in surgical failure.

Besides the obvious, there are certain other properties root-end filling materials must possess to be a material of choice, as quoted by Shin et al. in 2017:

1) Bacteriostatic or bactericidal
2) Dimensionally stable
3) Radiopaque
4) Noncorrosive
5) Resistant to dissolution
6) Dentinogenic, osteogenic, cementogenic
7) Adheres to tooth structure
8) Nonstaining to the teeth or tissue
9) Easy to manipulate [24]

Thus, the ideal properties should adhere to physical, biological, economic, and practical criteria.

4.5 Bioceramic Materials

Further in the chapter, we will discuss different bioceramic materials available, their composition, properties, contribution in periradicular surgery as root-end filling material, and their impact on surrounding tissues (Table 4.1).

4.5.1 Mineral Trioxide Aggregate

Dr. Torabinejad developed MTA from Portland cement (gray powder) that was marketed as ProRoot MTA, following which, to resolve the aesthetic concerns,

Table 4.1   Below is a table listing the most commonly available bioceramic cement for root-end filling material.

Product/manufacturer	Composition	Setting time
Grey ProRoot Mineral Trioxide Aggregate (G-MTA)	Powder: tricalcium silicate, dicalcium silicate, bismuth oxide, tricalcium aluminate, calcium sulfate dihydrate or gypsum, calcium aluminoferrite	165 min
Dentsply Tulsa Dental Specialties, Johnson City, USA	Liquid: water	
White ProRoot Mineral Trioxide Aggregate (W-MTA)	Powder: tricalcium silicate, dicalcium silicate, bismuth oxide, tricalcium aluminate, calcium sulfate dihydrate or gypsum	170 min
Dentsply Tulsa Dental Specialties, Johnson City, USA	Liquid: water	
Calcium-enriched mixture cement (CEM)	Powder: different compounds of calcium, including oxide, sulfate, phosphate, carbonate, silicate, hydroxide, and chloride compounds	50 min
Bionique Dent, Tehran, Iran	Liquid: water-based solution	
Biodentine	Powder: tricalcium silicate, dicalcium silicate, calcium carbonate, zirconium oxide, calcium oxide, iron oxide	45 min
Septodont, Saint-Maur-des-fossés, Cedex, France	Liquid: calcium chloride, a hydrosoluble (water-soluble) polymer, water.	
BioAggregate	Powder: tricalcium silicate, dicalcium silicate, tantalum pentoxide, calcium phosphate monobasic, amorphous silicon oxide	1260 min
Innovative Bioceramix, Vancouver, Canada	Liquid: deionized water	
EndoSequence Root Repair Material Putty and Paste (ERRM)	Calcium silicates, zirconium oxide, tantalum oxide, calcium phosphate monobasic and filler agents	4 h
Brasseler USA, Savannah, GA, USA		
iRoot BP Plus Root Repair Material (BP-RRM)	Calcium silicates, zirconium oxide, tantalum oxide/pentoxide, calcium phosphate monobasic	2 h (The manufacturer)
Innovative Bioceramix, Vancouver, Canada		

Source: Abusrewil et al. [13]/with permission of Elsevier.

white MTA, a tooth-colored formulation was introduced. Gray MTA comprises tricalcium silicate, tricalcium aluminate, tricalcium oxide silicate oxide, mineral oxide, and bismuth oxide (incorporated to make it more radiopaque). White MTA varies from gray MTA because of the lack of iron. The initial setting time is stated to be 4 hours; however, permanent setting requires at least 48 hours.

As mentioned earlier, MTA in comparison to amalgam, SuperEBA, and IRM is more resistant to bacterial contamination and fluid penetration. Recent studies reveal that when MTA comes into contact with tissue fluid, a layer of hydroxyapatite (HA) forms on the surface (also known as biomineralization) during its setting period, which is responsible for a biological seal between MTA and the dentin interface. According to histological studies, it was observed that MTA showed nearly negligible signs of inflammation when tested as a root-end filling material in an animal model. As per a study conducted at the University of Pennsylvania on a dog model, new cementum-like and bone-like growth was observed atop an MTA root-end filling (Figure 4.1). Varied in vitro cell cultures exhibited significant cell growth and attachments of several cells such as DPSC, human cementum-derived cells, mouse primary osteoblasts, MDPC23, etc., thereby showcasing a positive biocompatibility profile (Figure 4.2). The high pH of MTA facilitates hard

(a)   (b)

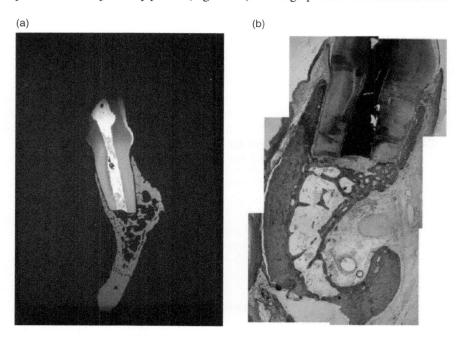

Figure 4.1 The pictures below demonstrate the root apex of a dog with ProRoot MTA. (a) Micro Computer Tomography. (b) Histological section. *Source:* Shin et al. [24]/with permission from John Wiley & Sons.

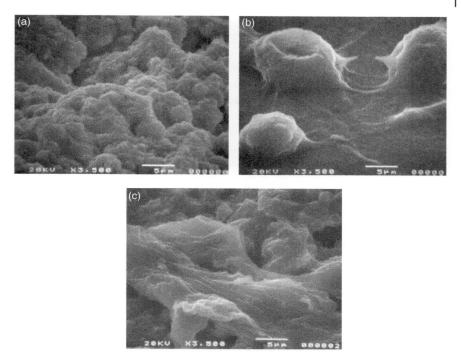

Figure 4.2 Pictures under the scanning electron microscope of MDPC23 cells on (a) a plastic plate. (b) and (c) ProRoot MTA; showcasing the cell growth on the same under high magnification. *Source:* Shin et al. [24]/with permission from John Wiley & Sons.

tissue formation or, more specifically, aids in tertiary dentin formation; thus, it suffices the criteria of being dentinogenic, osteogenic, and cementogenic. However, MTA comes with its share of drawbacks as well; for example, the probability of staining the remaining tooth structure, prolonged setting time, difficulty in the placement of MTA after retrograde cavity preparation, and so on. [24].

Several modifications of MTA have been brought into the scenario such as MTABio, MTA Angelus, OrthoMTA, and EndoCem MTA. However, more research is required to substantiate their uses in clinical practice [24].

4.5.2 Bioaggregate

MTA monopolized the research into root-end filling materials for almost a decade until a new bioceramic cement called BioAggregate (calcium silicate–based cement). It was introduced by Bioceramics Inc. in 2006 and was promoted by DiaDent as DiaRoot. Leal et al. in a study concluded that there was no difference, when it came to leakage in retrograde cavities, between MTA and

BioAggregate; both materials are equally noncytotoxic [25]. Like MTA, BioAggregate is also mixed from powder and liquid, deionized water is also provided with the same.

Personal preference dictates the preferred root-end filling material between MTA or BioAggregate because both are expected to perform well. Although in the root tip, aesthetics is not an area of concern, in regions where it is, BioAggregate or Biodentine can be used as opposed to MTA. Keskin et al. deduced that the color stability of different calcium silicate-based materials, when exposed to different irrigating solutions, was better in materials free of bismuth oxide [26].

4.5.3 Biodentine

Septodont introduced Biodentine in 2011 as a material that could be a replacement for dentin. In contrast to MTA, which showed mild to negligent reaction, Mori et al. stated that Biodentine exhibited moderated inflammation of the tissue on the seventh day. However, on the 14th day, both materials exhibited the same level of mild inflammation [27]. A lot of research proves microleakage with Biodentine is much less as compared to other materials. According to Grech et al., when compared to BioAggregate, Biodentine exhibited a high washout, thereby inferring that Biodentine filling must be protected while rinsing the retrograde cavity [28].

4.5.4 iRoot BP Plus Bioceramic Putty

This material is a water-based bioceramic synthesized purely in the laboratory. Because it is available in a premixed hydraulic formula, it is fairly easy and convenient to use. A recent study on the cytotoxic profile of iRoot BP concluded that it was as biocompatible as MTA and does not incite critical cytotoxicity [14].

4.5.5 Capasio

Capasio (Primus Consulting, Bradenton, FL), a recently developed calcium aluminosilicate-based material has been established in an attempt to enhance the shortcomings of preceding materials. Primarily composed of dental glass, bismuth oxide, and calcium aluminosilicate with a water-based gel, its powder is mixed with its gel and liquid in a 4 : 1 ratio by weight [29]. This is moderately more acidic (pH = 10.9) than WMTA (pH = 11.6) when finally set at nine minutes. Besides, it has exhibited analogous or improved physical characteristics including radiopacity, compressive strength, setting time, washout resistance, and pH [29]. It has been noted that Capasio is more likely to enter dentinal tubules when used as a root-end filling material because all its particles are less than 20 mm, with a mean particle size of 5.3 mm and, much like MTA, on exposure to synthetic tissue fluid it encouraged apatite deposition [30]. However, in contrast to MTA and Generex A, Capasio has not been demonstrated to boost primary osteoblast growth or promote nodule formation in a comparative analysis [31].

4.5.6 Calcium-Enriched Material

Calcium-enriched material (CEM) cement was first established in 2006 by Asgary et al. and is regarded to have great similarity to MTA, besides improved physical properties. The major and minor components of the powder in the descending order of their percentage weight include 51.75% wt. calcium oxide (CaO), 9.53% wt. sulfur trioxide (SO_3), 8.49% wt. phosphorous pentoxide (P_2O_5), 6.32% wt. silicon dioxide (SiO_2), aluminum trioxide (Al_2O_3), sodium aluminum oxide (Na_2O), magnesium oxide (MgO), and chloride (Cl), 23.91% wt. respectively [32]. It creates a bioactive calcium and phosphate-enhanced mixture when combined with a water-based solution showing alkaline pH of 10.71 ± 0.19 and a setting time of about 50 minutes [33]. In addition to creating HA in simulated bodily tissue fluid, mixed CEM cement also does so in ordinary saline solution, the latter of which differs from MTA [34]. Additionally, the calcium and phosphorus ions that are released by this innovative cement from indigenous sources create a rich pool of hydroxyl (OH), phosphate (PO^4) ions, and calcium (Ca^{2+}), which are ultimately utilized in the synthesis of HA [35]. It should be noted that other biomaterials in normal saline solution do not exhibit this effect. When CEM is established, its small expansion, suitable flow, and film thickness (increased flow and decreased film thickness) can guarantee a strong seal and minimize any subsequent leakage, as well as having the capacity to encourage cementogenesis over both the material and dentinal surface at the root-end. A noteworthy characteristic is the presence of entrapped cementocytes and insertions of periodontal ligament fibers in the newly produced eosinophilic cementum [36]. Another important feature is uninterrupted cementum covering across the root-end filling and the surrounding dentin; this can act as a safeguard against the potentially harmful residual material inside the root canal system. The similarity between the calcium, phosphorus, and oxygen distribution patterns on the surface of CEM cement and the surrounding dentin is yet another characteristic that may be helpful in tissue regeneration [37]. In dry, blood-contaminated, and saliva-contaminated conditions, Hasheminia et al.'s [38] assessment of the sealing performance of MTA and CEM cement as root-end filling materials revealed that CEM cement performed better. Studies have been conducted to compare the sealing capabilities of MTA and IRM with CEM cement which demonstrated that

CEM has a better sealing capacity than MTA and IRM. Its handling features and chemical properties could be the cause of the exceptional sealing. The capacity of CEM to release calcium ions during setting and the subsequent binding of calcium with phosphorus to produce HA crystals have both been linked to the material's biocompatibility. More than a shift in permeability, which promotes healing, this new biomaterial is more likely to result in changes pertaining to cellular enzymatic activity [37, 39]. Using an enzyme-linked immunosorbent assay and an MTT experiment, Mozayeni et al. assessed the cytotoxicity of CEM cement in comparison to MTA and IRM on mouse fibroblasts. CEM cement showed superior cell vitality versus MTA and IRM [40]. In a recent study, it was determined by histological analysis that in contrast to CEM cement, MTA causes cellular necrosis. The existence of dystrophic calcification close to the biomaterials was another significant discovery [32]. It is believed that a combination of properties, including sealing ability, biocompatibility, high alkalinity, antimicrobial action, HA formation, and similarity to dentin, cause CEM cement to induce the formation of hard tissue in the body [41]. Direct and indirect pulp capping, pulpotomy, furcation perforation repair, apexification, root resorption repair, and apexogenesis are some of its further applications [32]. In their prospective trial from 2013, Asgary and Ehsani (2013) reported a 1.5-year follow-up observation with a 93% overall success rate [42].

4.5.7 EndoSequence

An additional bioactive substance that is hydrophilic, extremely radiopaque, dimensionally stable, and generates HA upon setting is EndoSequence BC sealer (Brasseler, USA). It is a substance whose setting reaction requires the natural canal moisture found in the dentinal tubule. It is a premixed calcium silicate (CS) that may be handled with greater ease than MTA because it comes in the form of a syringeable paste or putty. It contains filler, thickening agents, CSs, calcium phosphate monobasic, zirconium oxide, and calcium hydroxide [43]. The material, according to the manufacturer, is devoid of aluminum, less soluble, and more dimensionally stable while setting [44]. It is a radiopaque material with a two- to four-hour setting time [45]. In the presence of environmental moisture, microhardness decreases while the premature setting accelerates [46]. In terms of dimensional accuracy, solubility, and film thickness, it complies with the International Organization for Standardization (ISO). Because of its nanoparticles, it can enter dentinal tubules. Upon setting, dentin liquid will form a mechanical link with the substance. Less shrinkage occurs, as a result, maintaining dimensional stability [47]. EndoSequence can seal just as well as MTA when employed as root-end infill material [48]. It develops a surface layer of HA when in contact with saliva [49]. Calcium release causes the deposition of hard tissue because of the alkaline pH, and due to its high pH, it also exhibits antibacterial activity against *Enterococcus faecalis* [50].

4.5.8 EndoBinder

A new calcium aluminate–based endodontic cement (Patent Number PI07045026, 2007) named EndoBinder (Binderware, São Carlos, SP, Brazil) has been developed at the Federal University of São Carlos, with the goal of maintaining the characteristics and clinical applications of MTA while removing its unfavorable traits. It is composed of (% by weight) Al_2O_3 (68.5), CaO (#31.0), SiO_2 (0.3–0.8), MgO (0.4–0.5), and Fe_2O_3 (<0.3) that has appropriate biological and antimicrobial capabilities, according to Pandolfelli et al. [51] and Jacobovitz et al. [52]. The procedure of calcining Al_2O_3 and $CaCO_3$ at temperatures between 1315 and 1425 °C, which is the most practical way to generate materials with a more consistent composition, is used to create cement. After cooling, the calcium aluminate is triturated until the desired particle size is attained. The following chemical reaction can serve as a general description of how EndoBinder is created: $CaCO_3 + Al_2O_3 = Ca(AlO_2)_2 + CO_2$. In comparison to MTA, the EndoBinder laboratory synthesis process offers several benefits, including better control of impurity levels, particularly Fe_2O_3, which promotes tooth staining [53, 54], and free MgO and CaO, which cause an unintended expansion of the material when they come into contact with moisture [55]. Greater compatibility between living tissues and cement is encouraged by the balance between stoichiometric phases rich in Al_2O_3 and CaCO3, which is responsible for the hydrophilic setting process of EndoBinder, as well as sufficient physicochemical characteristics [56, 57]. When it comes to the material's biocompatibility and physicomechanical qualities, the balance between phases rich in Al_2O_3 and $CaCO_3$ that EB permits produce better results [56, 57]. It typically consists of three primary stoichiometric phases: the anhydrous phase CA ($CaO.Al_2O_3$), which accounts for between 40 and 70% of the product; the CA2 ($CaO.2Al_2O_3$) phase, which is ranked second in proportion (25%); and the $C_{12}A_7$ ($12CaO.7Al_2O_3$) phase, which accounts for 10%. The growth of the crystals present in the phases known as calcium aluminate hydrates occurs after this process has continued until the solution reaches a sufficient level of saturation to encourage its precipitation [58]. Because of the equilibrium allowed between phases rich in Al_2O_3 and CaCO3, the hydrated phases precipitated establish strong connections between the particles that make up the cement, characterizing its setting and giving the material mechanical strength and biological tolerance concerning living tissues [51, 58, 59]. This balance minimizes the addition of additives to the cement's original formulation and permits control over the setting time [51, 58]. In turn, the faster setting time ensures superior clinical application conditions for the cement and reduces its oral solubility and disintegration [51, 60]. As a result, it was shown that EB was biocompatible and displayed less tissue reactivity than MTA when tested in rat subcutaneous tissue. Tests on rat subcutaneous tissue revealed that it is biocompatible and that MMP-2 and MMP-9 did not exhibit any gelatinolytic activity [61]. This material is known to have adequate physical and mechanical properties [62] and good cell responsiveness, allowing for more cell development at an advanced stage of osteoblastic differentiation than was possible with MTA [63]. Garcia et al. claim that EB has a more uniform microstructural arrangement than MTA, with globular particles that are similar in size and shape allowing for better cement flow and stress distribution, which may have been key to the maximum bond strength seen in this research. The compressive and diametral tensile strength tests produced exceptional results [64]. Recent studies have also demonstrated good biological properties in vitro and in vivo, tissue biocompatibility, and lack of MMP-2 gelatinolytic activity in relation to EndoBinder [57, 65]. This constant release of calcium ions causes the cement to gradually raise the pH of the medium, which reaches its maximum level in about 30 days [65], which is the time frame in which it is possible to observe a significant number of osteogenic cells acting in linear closure of the bone defects in the current study.

4.5.9 Generex A

Generex A is a CS-based substance particularly produced with powder components that are finer than those in white MTA, but it is blended with special gels as opposed to the water used in MTA. Compared to MTA, Generex A material has better handling characteristics [29]. It is generally composed of bismuth oxide, tricalcium aluminate, dicalcium silicate, and tricalcium silicate with a mixing gel including sodium lauryl sulfate and additional unidentified chemicals, in accordance with the material safety data sheet [66]. Generex A is easy to form into a rope-like mass comparable to IRM because it combines to a dough-like consistency [29]. To nucleate the formation of HA in vivo, the Generex A powder contains HA, and for radiopacity it contains bismuth oxide[1]. Generex A components contain HA, which could speed up osteoblast activity. The powders for the Generex A and Capasio materials include CS among others, and it was anticipated that during the setting reactions, calcium hydroxide would also be released. Apatite is probably the dominant calcium phosphate phase that precipitates on the surface of such objects when the phosphate-containing solution's pH surpasses 9.25 [67]. The fact that water is a component of the liquid or gel used to set the powders gave the experimental materials exceptional resilience to washout and made them appropriate for moist environments. Osteoblasts were able to attach and multiply on both MTA and Generex A materials in this study [66], but only MTA promoted nodule development as documented by Perez et al. [63] and Danesh et al. [68] On Generex A, no nodule formation was seen, although there was a layering of cells, which often comes before nodule formation. Of the materials examined, Generex A was the most biocompatible, enabling rat osteoblasts to adhere and multiply similarly to MTA. Generex A may be a suitable reparative material for endodontics given its better handling characteristics [66].

4.5.10 Quick-Set

The cationic surfactant from the liquid gel component of Capasio powder was eliminated because it was believed to affect its biocompatibility, and the powder was refined and given the name Quick-Set (Primus Consulting) [66]. Quick-Set showed comparable in vitro cytotoxicity profiles to WMTA, according to recent biocompatibility research using a mouse dental papilla-derived odontoblast-like cell line (MDPC-23) (conducted with methylthiazol diphenyltetrazolium test, vital cell staining, and flow cytometry) [69]. After the elution of their cytotoxic components, Quick-Set and MTA have similar in vitro osteogenic/dentogenic differentiation capabilities [70]. In addition to the calcium mono- and dialuminate phases, the Quick-Set2 hybrid cement (Primus Consulting, Bradenton, FL, USA) even has a silicate phase. These hybrid cements have short setting times and acid resistance thanks to the aluminate phases, while the silicate component aids in mineralogic reactions. Free bismuth oxide and alumina (Al_2O_3) that were existing in the prior Quick-Set material have been removed in this experimental substance. The percentage of the hydraulic phase increases in the absence of free alumina. The justification for eliminating free alumina is per the findings of earlier canine research using in vivo pulpotomy and root-end filling that suggested free alumina could provide irrigation to critical tissues [71, 72]. To distinguish from dentin, Quick-Set2 contains a radiopaque powder. The possibility of discoloration is eliminated in Quick-Set2 by replacing the bismuth oxide radiopacifier with tantalum pentoxide (Ta_2O_5) [73]. A recent study [73] reported on the biocompatibility of Quick-Set2 calcium aluminosilicate cement. After two cycles of aging in deionized water, there were no changes in cytotoxicity between the control (tricalcium silicate cement) and the experimental material. When both types of cement were used in the close interface to undifferentiated human dental pulp stem cells, they were less cytotoxic than cement composed of zinc oxide and eugenol (hDPSCs). The osteogenic capacity of hDPSCs is enhanced by Quick-Set2, with the former showing stronger effects. Additional research utilizing in vivo animal models is necessary to confirm the potential enhancing osteogenic effects of the experimental discoloration-free calcium aluminosilicate cement. Quick-Set2 is said to offer comparable short setting times, ultimate pH, acid resistance, tubule penetration, and washout resistance to its forerunners, Quick-Set and Capasio [29, 31, 73]. Quick-Set has exhibited enhanced healing and osteogenic/dentinogenic qualities in vivo animal models, while in vitro tests have revealed that Quick-Set and Quick-Set2 are equally as biocompatible as ProRoot MTA [70, 74–76]. Additionally, ProRoot MTA and Quick-Set have comparable in vitro osteogenic/dentinogenic characteristics [70]. A radiopacifier, calcium aluminosilicate powder, and other proprietary ingredients are combined with a special water-based gel to create Quick-Set2. To prevent tooth discoloration brought on by the presence of bismuth oxide, which is contained in ProRoot MTA and some other MTA-type materials, Quick-Set2 incorporates tantalum oxide, just like NeoMTA Plus [77]. Additionally, compared to Quick-predecessors, Set2's Capasio, and Quick-Set, Quick-Set2 has fewer loose alumina particles.

4.5.11 Ceramicrete-D

Ceramicrete-D has been established because of its possible bioactivity, significantly greater sealing power than white ProRoot MTA (Dentsply Tulsa Dental Specialties, Tulsa, OK), and pH that is basic after setting [1]. Despite having extended final set periods (>one hour), the novel materials were simple to use and unresponsive to rinsing, which suggests that the working time (initial set time) was substantially shorter. A prior investigation demonstrated that when immersed in deionized water or a fluid containing phosphate, set Ceramicrete-D produced an alkaline (pH of about 11 after 72 hours) [67]. This significant variation suggests that longer-term pH assessments of specified samples in water are crucial to comprehending the performance of promising materials. In a phosphate-buffered solution, Ceramicrete-D has already been demonstrated to cause hydroxyl-apatite precipitation. As water is a component of the gel or liquid used to set the powders, the clinical handling of these root-end filling materials was superior to WMTA. They also showed outstanding washout resistance and were ideal for damp situations. Modifications to the recipe should boost the strength and radiopacity of Ceramicrete-D. An acid phosphate and a tiny amount of soluble basic metal oxide undergo an acid-base reaction to generate the self-setting phosphate ceramic known as Ceramicrete, which sets in ambient conditions (calcined MgO). More recently, cerium oxide radiopaque filler and hydroxyapatite powder were added to phosphosilicate ceramic to create a biocompatible, radiopaque dental material. The initial setting time for the Ceramicrete-based material is 6 minutes, and the ultimate setting time is 12 minutes. It also sets underwater with little washout and may be twisted into a sausage shape for easy manipulation with dental tools. By combining the powder with deionized water, a modified version of the Ceramicrete-D was introduced. According to reports, Ceramicrete-D can be sealed well. Two endodontic biocer-amic repair cement (BioAggregate and Ceramicrete-D) showed comparable leak-age results to white MTA when employed as root-end filling materials in a different study by Leal et al. [25] Glucose penetration was considerably decreased in Ceramicrete-D. Physical and chemical investigations revealed that Ceramicrete-D had better clinical handling and washout resistance than MTA, but that it was less radiopaque, less robust, and more acidic at first than Capasio and Generex A [78].

4.5.12 Bioglass

Bioglass (BG) includes the glass type of $Na_2O-CaO-SiO_2-P_2O_5$ in a predeter-mined ratio [79], with silica (SiO_2) making up around 50% of the total composi-tion [79, 80]. For many years, orthopedic surgery has used BG in clinical settings. When BG is inserted in a defect area near the bone, reactions on the BG surface cause the release of essential amounts of soluble Ca, Si, P, and Na ions, which stimulate favorable intra- and extracellular responses and hasten bone forma-tion [81]. After this bone development, the silica-rich gel begins to form on the BG surface. When ions from physiological fluids interact with silica-rich gel, hydroxyapatite (HA)-like material is created on the surface of the BG. Additionally, in the silica-rich gel, osteoblasts create new bone, which enables BG to connect to the bone via the synthesis of bone-like HA layers and biological interactions with collagen [82, 83]. Additionally, BG can encourage bone cells to renew and recover on their own, greatly increasing the kinetics of tissue healing [81]. The terms "osteoconductivity" and "osteoinductivity" refer to these characteris-tics [84, 85]. Although BG has mostly been used in applications where it comes in touch with bone tissue, it has lately shown promise in triggering the regenera-tion of soft tissues as well [86, 87]. Since its ionic dissolution products were dis-covered to induce angiogenesis, BG has piqued the curiosity of numerous researchers. There are currently additional BG-based products available for use in peripheral nerve regeneration and wound repair [88]. These uses imply that BG exhibits adaptability and biocompatibility as a biomaterial capable of being applied to both soft tissues such as dental pulp and periapical tissue and hard tissues such as cementum or dentin because these materials resemble the bone [89].

Table 4.2 below depicts the outcome in terms of the success rate of peri-radicular surgeries with various root-end filling materials.

Table 4.2 The success rate of peri-radicular surgeries with various root-end filling materials.

Authors	Year	Study design	Number of teeth	Root-end filling material	Follow-up observation	Overall success rate
Asgary and Ehsani	2013	Prospective study	13	Calcium enriched mixture (CEM)	1.5 years	93%
Çalışkan et al.	2016	Clinical study	90	ProRoot MTA	2–6 years	80%
Jing et al.	2012	Clinical study	54	MTA	1 year	92.6%
Kim et al.	2016	Randomised controlled study	182	MTA and SuperEBA	4 years	91.6 and 89.9% respectively
Saunders	2008	Prospective study	276	ProRoot White MTA	3 years	88.8%
Shen et al.	2016	Prospective study	97	MTA	1 year	92.8%
Shinbori et al.	2015	Retrospective study	113	EndoSequence BC Root Repair (ERRM)	1 year	92%
Song and Kim	2012	Prospective randomized controlled study	192	MTA and SuperEBA	1 year	95.6 and 93.1% respectively
Von Arx et al.	2010	Prospective study	353	ProRoot MTA and Retroplast	1 year	91.3 and 79.5% respectively
	2014		271		5 years	92.5 and 76.6% respectively
Von Arx et al.	2007	Cohort study	191	ProRoot MTA, SuperEBA or Retroplast	1 year	90.2, 76.4 and 84.7% respectively (86.4%), 67.3 and 75.3% respectively
	2012		170		5 years	
Wang et al.	2017	Prospective cohort study	74	ProRoot MTA	1–2.5 years	90.5%
Zhou et al.	2017	Prospective randomized controlled study	158	MTA and iRoot BP Plus Root Repair Material (BP-RRM).	1 year	93.1 and 94.4%, respectively

Source: Abusrewil et al. [13]/with permission of Elsevier.

4.6 Conclusion

With the introduction of the first bioceramic material MTA in the 1990s, a plethora of new bioceramic cement appeared in an era of ultrasonic devices and microscopes, which were specifically developed to facilitate procedures including retrograde cavity preparation. Not only as retrograde fillings, bioceramics have also found their place in other treatment modalities, e.g. regenerative endodontics, open apex cases, vital pulp therapy, and perforation repairs.

Bioceramics have shown superior and promising results as compared to traditional materials like amalgam, IRM, SuperEBA, etc. Although, without a doubt, bioceramic materials are one of the best options available today for root-end filling because of their biocompatibility, antimicrobial profile, bioactivity, and ability to impart long-term seal, their relative importance is yet to be explored and has to be supported with long-term clinical research to justify the in vitro findings. Therefore, before reaching to any concrete coclusion, furthur reasearch is required to establish the superior performance of endodontic bioceramics in comparison to other endodontic materials.

References

1 Rhodes, J.S. (2006). *Advanced Endodontics: Clinical Retreatment and Surgery*, 147–148. CRC Press.
2 Carrotte, P. (2011). A clinical guide to endodontics. *British Dental Association* 80–84.
3 Gatewood, R.S. (2007). Endodontic materials. *Dental Clinics of North America* 51 (3): 695–712.
4 Torabinejad, M. and Walton, R.E. (2009). *Endodontics: Principles and Practice*. Saunders.
5 Ørstavik, D. (2005). Materials used for root canal obturation: technical, biological and clinical testing. *Endodontic Topics* 12: 25–38.
6 Grossman, L.I. (1978). *Endodontic Practice*. Philadelphia: Lea & Febiger.
7 Pitt, L.S.W. (1982). Endodontic filling materials. In: *Biocompatibility of Dental Materials* (ed. D.C. Smith and D.F. Williams), 223–257. Boca Raton: CRC Press.
8 Spangberg, L., Engström, B., and Langeland, K. (1973). Biologic effects of dental materials. 3. Toxicity and antimicrobial effect of endodontic antiseptics in vitro. *Oral Surgery, Oral Medicine, and Oral Pathology* 36: 856–871.
9 Pitt Ford, T.R. (1991). Endodontic materials and techniques. *Current Opinion in Dentistry* 1: 729–733.
10 Hauman, C.H. and Love, R.M. (2003). Biocompatibility of dental materials used in contemporary endodontic therapy: a review. Part 1. Intracanal drugs and substances. *International Endodontic Journal* 36: 75–85.

11 Hauman, C.H. and Love, R.M. (2003). Biocompatibility of dental materials used in contemporary endodontic therapy: a review. Part 2. Root-canal-filling materials. *International Endodontic Journal* 36: 147–160.

12 Haapasalo, M., Parhar, M., Huang, X. et al. (2015). Clinical use of bioceramic materials. *Endodontic Topics* 32 (1): 97–117.

13 Abusrewil, S.M., McLean, W., and Scott, J.A. (2018). The use of bioceramics as root-end filling materials in periradicular surgery: a literature review. *The Saudi Dental Journal* 30 (4): 273–282.

14 Saxena, P., Gupta, S.K., and Newaskar, V. (2013). Biocompatibility of root – end filling materials: recent update. *Restorative Dentistry Endodontics* 38 (3): 119–127.

15 Vasudev, S., Goel, B., and Tyagi, S. (2003). Root end filling materials – a review. *Endodontology* 15: 12–18.

16 Marti-Bowen, E., Penarrocha-Diago, M., and García-Mira, B. (2004). Periapical surgery using the ultrasound technique and silver amalgam retrograde filling. A study of 71 teeth with 100 canals. *Medicina Oral, Patología Oral y Cirugía Bucal* 10: E67–E73.

17 Crosher, R., Dinsdale, R., and Holmes, A. (1989). A one visit apicectomy technique using calcium hydroxide cement as the canal filling material combined with retrograde amalgam. *International Endodontic Journal* 22 (6): 283–289.

18 Gartner, A. and Dorn, S. (1992). Advances in endodontic surgery. *Dental Clinics of North America* 36 (2): 357–378.

19 Amagasa, T., Nagase, M., Sato, T., and Shioda, S. (1989). Apicoectomy with retrograde gutta-percha root filling. *Oral Surgery, Oral Medicine, and Oral Pathology* 68 (3): 339–342.

20 Hendra, L.P. (1970). EBA cement. A practical system for all cementation. *International Endodontic Journal* 4 (2): 28–31.

21 Bondra, D.L., Hartwell, G.R., MacPherson, M.G., and Portell, F.R. (1989). Leakage in vitro with IRM, high copper amalgam, and EBA cement as retrofilling materials. *Journal of Endodontia* 15 (4): 157–160.

22 Koch, K.A. and Brave, D.G. (2012). Bioceramics, part 1: the clinician's viewpoint. *Dentistry Today* 31 (1): 130–135.

23 Torabinejad, M., Rastegar, A.F., Kettering, J.D., and Pitt Ford, T.R. (1995). Bacterial leakage of mineral trioxide aggregate as a root-end filling material. *Journal of Endodontia* 21: 109–112.

24 Shin, S., Chen, I., Karabucak, B. et al. (2017). MTA and bioceramic root end filling materials. In: *Microsurgery in Endodontics* (ed. S. Kim and S. Kratchman), 91–99. Wiley.

25 Leal, F., De-Deus, G., Brandão, C. et al. (2011). Comparison of the root-end seal provided by bioceramic repair cements and white MTA. *International Endodontic Journal* 44: 662–668.

26 Keskin, C., Demiryurek, E.O., and Ozyurek, T. (2015). Color stabilities of calcium silicate-based materials in contact with different irrigation solutions. *Journal of Endodontia* 41: 409–411.

27 Mori, G.G., Teixeira, L.M., de Oliveira, D.L. et al. (2014). Biocompatibility evaluation of biodentine in subcutaneous tissue of rats. *Journal of Endodontia* 40: 1485–1488.

28 Grech, L., Mallia, B., and Camilleri, J. (2013). Investigation of the physical properties of tricalcium silicate cement-based root-end filling materials. *Dental Materials* 29: e20–e28.

29 Porter, M.L., Berto, A., Primus, C.M., and Watanabe, I. (2010). Physical and chemical properties of new-generation endodontic materials. *Journal of Endodontia* 36: 524–528.

30 Parker, K.M. and Sharp, J.H. (1982). Refractory calcium aluminate cements. *Transactions and Journal of the British Ceramic Society* 81: 35–42.

31 Bird, D.C., Komabayashi, T., Guo, L. et al. (2012). In vitro evaluation of dentinal tubule penetration and biomineralization ability of a new root-end filling material. *Journal of Endodontia* 38 (8): 1093–1096.

32 Bali, P., Shivekshith, A.K., Allamaprabhu, C.R., and Vivek, H.P. (2014). Calcium enriched mixture cement: a review. *International Journal of Contemporary Dental and Medical Reviews* 2014: 1–3.

33 Bhatia, C., Chandak, M., Adwani, D. et al. (2015). Calcium enriched mixture cement. *International Journal of Dental and Health Sciences* 2 (4): 905–910.

34 Asgary, S., Eghbal, M.J., Parirokh, M., and Ghoddusi, J. (2009). Effect of two storage solutions on surface topography of two root-end fillings. *Australian Endodontic Journal* 35: 147–152.

35 Utneja, S., Nawal, R.R., Talwar, S., and Verma, M. (2014). Current perspectives of bio-ceramic technology in endodontics: calcium enriched mixture cement – review of its composition, properties and applications. *Restorative Dentistry & Endodontics* 39: 1–13.

36 Asgary, S., Eghbal, M., and Ehsani, S. (2010). Periradicular regeneration after endodontic surgery with calcium-enriched mixture cement in dogs. *Journal of Endodontia* 36: 837.

37 Asgary, S., Eghbal, M.J., Parirokh, M. et al. (2009). Comparison of mineral trioxide aggregate's composition with Portland cements and a new endodontic cement. *Journal of Endodontia* 35 (2): 243–250.

38 Hasheminia, M., Nejad, S.L., and Asgary, S. (2010). Sealing ability of MTA and CEM cement as root-end fillings of human teeth in dry, saliva or blood-contaminated conditions. *Iranian Endodontic Journal* 5 (4): 151.

39 Asgary, S., Shahabi, S., Jafarzadeh, T. et al. (2008). The properties of a new endodontic material. *Journal of Endodontia* 34: 990–993.

40 Mozayeni, M.A., Milani, A.S., Marvasti, L.A., and Asgary, S. (2012). Cytotoxicity of calcium enriched mixture cement compared with mineral trioxide aggregate and intermediate restorative material. *Australian Endodontic Journal* 38 (2): 70–75.

41 Utneja, S., Nawal, R.R., Talwar, S., and Verma, M. (2015). Current perspectives of bio-ceramic technology in endodontics: calcium enriched mixture cement-review of its composition, properties and applications. *Restorative Dentistry & Endodontics* 40 (1): 1–3.

42 Friedman, S. (2017). Prognosis of healing in treated teeth with endodontic infections. In: *Endodontic Microbiology* (ed. A.F. Fouad), 341–384. Hoboken, NJ: Wiley.

43 Asgary, S., Eghbal, M.J., Parirokh, M., and Torabzadeh, H. (2006). Sealing ability of three commercial mineral trioxide aggregates and an experimental root – end filling material. *Iranian Endodontics Journal* 1: 101–105.

44 Chang, J.W.W., Praisarnti, C., and Neelakantan, P. (2017). Increasing use of bioceramics in endodontics: a narrative review. *Oral Health* .

45 Candeiro, G.T., Correia, F.C., Duarte, M.A. et al. (2012). Evaluation of radiopacity, pH, release of calcium ions, and flow of a bioceramic root canal sealer. *Journal of Endodontia* 38: 842–845.

46 Loushine, B.A., Bryan, T.E., Looney, S.W. et al. (2011). Setting properties and cytotoxicity evaluation of a premixed bioc eramic root c anal sealer. *Journal of Endodontia* 37: 673–677.

47 Zhou, H.M., Shen, Y., Zheng, W. et al. (2013). Physical properties of 5 root canal sealers. *Journal of Endodontia* 39: 1281–1286.

48 Shokouhinejad, N., Nekoofar, M.H., Ashoftehyazdi, K. et al. (2014). Marginal adaptation of new bioceramic materials and mineral trioxide aggregate: a scanning electron microscopy study. *Iranian Endodontics Journal* 9: 144–148.

49 Shokouhinejad, N., Nekoofar, M.H., Razmi, H. et al. (2012). Bioactivity of EndoSequence root repair material and bioaggregate. *International Endodontic Journal* 45: 1127–1134.

50 Lovato, K.F. and Sedgley, C.M. (2011). Antibacterial activity of endosequence root repair material and proroot MTA against clinical isolates of Enterococcus faecalis. *Journal of Endodontia* 37: 1542–1546.

51 Pandolfelli VC, Oliveira IR, Rosseto HL, and Jacobovitz M. (2007). A composition based on aluminate cement for application in endodontics and the obtained cement product. Patent registration INPI 0704502-6, Portuguese.

52 Jacobovitz, M., Vianna, M.E., Pandolfelli, V.C. et al. (2009). Root canal filling with cements based on mineral aggregates: an in vitro analysis of bacterial microleakage. *Oral Surgery, Oral Medicine, Oral Pathology, Oral Radiology, and Endodontics* 108: 140–144.

53 Jacobovitz, M. and de Lima, R.K. (2008). Treatment of inflammatory internal root resorption with mineral trioxide aggregate: a case report. *International Endodontic Journal* 41: 905–912.

54 Garcia Lda, F., Aguilar, F.G., Rossetto, H.L. et al. (2013). Staining susceptibility of new calcium aluminate cement (EndoBinder) in teeth: a 1-year in vitro study. *Dental Traumatology* 29: 383–388.

55 Kazemi, R.B., Safavi, K.E., and Sp_angberg LS. (1993). Dimensional changes of endodontic sealers. *Oral Surgery, Oral Medicine, and Oral Pathology* 76: 766–771.

56 Bortoluzzi, E.A., Broon, N.J., Bramante, C.M. et al. (2006). Sealing ability of MTA and radiopaque Portland cement with or without calcium chloride for root-end filling. *Journal of Endodontia* 32: 897–900.

57 Aguilar, F.G., Roberti Garcia, L.F., and Panzeri Pires-de-Souza, F.C. (2012). Biocompatibility of new calcium aluminate cement (EndoBinder). *Journal of Endodontia* 38: 367–371.

58 Oliveira, I.R., Pandolfelli, V.C., and Jacobovitz, M. (2010). Chemical, physical and mechanical properties of a novel calcium aluminate endodontic cement. *International Endodontic Journal* 43: 1069–1076.

59 Castro-Raucci, L.M., Oliveira, I.R., Teixeira, L.N. et al. (2011). Effects of a novel calcium aluminate cement on the early events of the progression of osteogenic cell cultures. *Brazilian Dental Journal* 22: 99–104.

60 Hammad, M., Qualtrough, A., and Silikas, N. (2008). Extended setting shrinkage behavior of endodontic sealers. *Journal of Endodontia* 34: 90–93.

61 Silva, E.J., Accorsi-Mendonça, T., Almeida, J.F. et al. (2012). Evaluation of cytotoxicity and up-regulation of gelatinases in human fibroblast cells by four root canal sealers. *International Endodontic Journal* 45 (1): 49–56.

62 Garcia, L.F., Aguilar, F.G., Sabino, M.G. et al. (2011). Mechanical and microstructural characterisation of new calcium aluminate cement (EndoBinder). *Advances in Applied Ceramics* 110: 469–475.

63 Perez, A.L., Spears, R., Gutmann, J.L., and Opperman, L.A. (2003). Osteoblasts and MG-63 osteosarcoma cells behave differently when in contact with ProRoot MTA and White MTA. *International Endodontic Journal* 36: 564–570.

64 Locher, F.W., Sprung, S., and Korf, P. (1973). Effect of the particle size distribution on the strength of Portland cement. *ZKG International* 26: 349–355.

65 Silva, E.J., Herrera, D.R., Almeida, J.F. et al. (2012). Evaluation of cytotoxicity and up-regulation of gelatinases in fibroblast cells by three root repair materials. *International Endodontic Journal* 45 (9): 815–820.

66 Washington, J.T., Schneiderman, E., Spears, R. et al. (2011). Biocompatibility and osteogenic potential of new generation endodontic materials established by using primary osteoblasts. *Journal of Endodontics* 37 (8): 1166–1170.

67 Tay, K.C., Loushine, B.A., Oxford, C. et al. (2007). In vitro evaluation of a ceramicrete-based rootend filling material. *Journal of Endodontia* 33: 1438–1443.

68 Danesh, F., Tootian, Z., Jahanbani, J. et al. (2010). Biocompatibility and mineralization activity of fresh or set white mineral trioxide aggregate, biomimetic carbonated apatite, and synthetic hydroxyapatite. *Journal of Endodontia* 36: 1036–1041.

69 Wei, W., Qi, Y.P., Nikonov, S.Y. et al. (2012). Effects of an experimental calcium aluminosilicate cement on the viability of murine odontoblast-like cells. *Journal of Endodontia* 38: 936–942.

70 Eid, A.A. et al. (2013). In vitro osteogenic/dentinogenic potential of an experimental calcium aluminosilicate cement. *Journal of Endodontics* 39 (9): 1161–1166. https://doi.org/10.1016/j.joen.2013.04.005.

71 Kohout, G.D., He, J., Primus, C.M. et al. (2015). Comparison of Quick-Set and mineral trioxide aggregate root-end fillings for the regeneration of apical tissues in dogs. *Journal of Endodontia* 41: 248–252.

72 Woodmansey, K.F., Kohout, G.D., Primus, C.M. et al. (2015). Histologic assessment of Quick-Set and mineral trioxide aggregate pulpotomies in a canine model. *Journal of Endodontia* 41: 1626–1630.

73 Niu, L.N., Watson, D., Thames, K. et al. (2015). Effects of a discoloration-resistant calcium aluminosilicate cement on the viability and proliferation of undifferentiated human dental pulp stem cells. *Scientific Reports* 5: 17177.

74 Cornelio, A.L., Rodrigues, E.M., Salles, L.P. et al. (2017). Bioactivity of MTA Plus, Biodentine and experimental calcium silicate-based cements in human osteoblast-like cells. *International Endodontic Journal* 50: 39–47.

75 Kramer, P.R., Woodmansey, K.F., White, R. et al. (2014). Capping a pulpotomy with calcium aluminosilicate cement: comparison to mineral trioxide aggregates. *Journal of Endodontia* 40: 1429–1434.

76 Niu, L.N., Pei, D.D., Morris, M. et al. (2016). Mineralogenic characteristics of osteogenic lineage-committed human dental pulp stem cells following their exposure to a discoloration-free calcium aluminosilicate cement. *Dental Materials* 32: 1235–1247.

77 Walsh, R.M., Woodmansey, K.F., He, J. et al. (2018). Histology of NeoMTA Plus and Quick-Set2 in contact with pulp and periradicular tissues in a canine model. *Journal of Endodontics* 44 (9): 1389–1395.

78 Raghavendra, S.S., Jadhav, G.R., Gathani, K.M., and Kotadia, P. (2017). Bioceramics in endodontics – a review. *Journal of Istanbul University Faculty of Dentistry* 51 (3 Suppl 1): S128–S137. https://doi.org/10.17096/jiufd.63659.

79 Hench, L.L. (2006). The story of Bioglass®. *Journal of Materials Science* 17: 967–978.

80 Jell, G. and Stevens, M.M. (2006). Gene activation by bioactive glasses. *Journal of Materials Science. Materials in Medicine* 17: 997–1002.

81 Xynos, I.D., Edgar, A.J., Buttery, L.D.K. et al. (2001). Gene expression profiling of human osteoblasts following treatment with the ionic products of Bioglass 45S5 dissolution. *Journal of Biomedical Materials Research* 55: 151–157.

82 Hench, L.L. (1991). Bioceramics: from concept to clinic. *Journal of the American Ceramic Society* 74: 1487–1510.

83 Hoeland, W., Vogel, W., Waumann, K., and Gummel, J. (1985). Interface reactions between machinable bioactive glass-ceramics and bone. *Journal of Biomedical Materials Research* 19: 303–312.

84 Hench, L.L. (2009). Genetic design of bioactive glass. *Journal of the European Ceramic Society* 29: 1257–1265.

85 Hench, L.L. and Polack, J.M. (2002). Third-generation biomedical materials. *Science* 295: 1014–1017.

86 Baino, F., Novajra, G., Miguez-Pacheco, V. et al. (2016). Bioactive glasses: special applications outside the skeletal system. *Journal of Non-Crystalline Solids* 432: 15–30.

87 Kokubo, T. and Takadama, H. (2006). How useful is SBF in predicting in vivo bone bioactivity? *Biomaterials* 27: 2907–2915.

88 Gilchrist, T., Glasby, M., Healy, D. et al. (1998). In vitro nerve repair-in vivo. The reconstruction of peripheral nerves by entubulation with biodegradable glass tubes – a preliminary report. *British Journal of Plastic Surgery* 51: 231–237.

89 Oguntebi, B., Clark, A., and Wilsin, J. (1993). Pulp capping with bioglass and autologous demineralized dentin in miniature swine. *Journal of Dental Research* 72: 484–489.

5

Bioceramics as an Apical Plug

Riccardo Tonini[1] and Marilu' Garo[2]

[1] *Department of Medical and Surgery Specialties, Radiological Sciences and Public Health, Dental School, University of Brescia, Brescia, Italy*
[2] *Mathsly Research, Vibo Valentia, Italy*

CONTENTS

5.1 Apical Plug

Endodontic treatment of teeth with immature root apices and necrotic pulp has always been challenging [1]. The risk of not sealing the root canal correctly, together with the high risk of inadequate root canal instrumentation and failure to achieve an adequate apical stop [2], has led scientific research to identify techniques and materials that can increase the success rate without sacrificing the balance between time and success, typical characteristics of endodontic practice.

Apexification, a traditional procedure for immature, nonvital teeth, is a method for inducing a calcified barrier in a root with an open apex or for further apical development of teeth with incomplete roots and necrotic pulp [3]. Apical plug, also known as one-step apexification, is an appropriate technique for immature teeth with pulp necrosis to create an apical barrier and achieve adequate stopping. Together with revitalization, it represents a therapeutic approach for eliminating signs and symptoms of infection and preserving affected teeth in the long term [4]. For many years, calcium hydroxide (CH) has been proposed as a successful material for the formation of a calcified barrier [5]. Although this material is effective and provides predictable results owing to its ability to form a calcified tissue at the root end, it has several disadvantages, such as the need for multiple sessions requiring high patient compliance, the high susceptibility of the tooth to fracture given the thin and fragile roots often characteristic of teeth with incomplete roots [6], the vulnerability of the provisional coronal restoration to re-infection [7], the long-term duration of CH use, which has been shown to weaken the tooth and increase the likelihood of dental fractures [8–12], and the long time required to form the calcified apical barrier (approximately six months) [13], as well as the nature of the barrier which is calcified but porous and sometimes contains a small amount of soft tissue.

Therefore, this technique has been replaced by a more powerful approach based on hydraulic calcium silicate cement, which reduces the treatment time to one or two visits, the risk of poor patient compliance, and root fractures. Mineral trioxide aggregate (MTA), used initially for root-end fillings and mainly composed of tricalcium silicate, tricalcium aluminate, tricalcium oxide, and silica, is a powder of fine hydrophilic particles which form a colloidal gel that solidifies into a rigid structure [6]. MTA is considered an optimal allay for the application of the apical plug technique. It offers many advantages, such as the ability to cure even in the presence of blood, a high pH (10.2–12.5 three hours after setting) [6], and can be used as an apical plug in immature, nonvital teeth because of its ability to form a cementitious tissue in the periradicular area of the tooth [6]. Overall, using MTA as an apical plug simplifies the complex procedure and promotes hard tissue, resulting in a biological seal of the cementum over the material [14].

In contrast to CH, MTA showed less inflammation and more hard tissue formation [15], whereas MTA is more effective when combined with an intracanal combination of CH for one week [16]. In addition, MTA has a good sealing ability, can be packed with a carrier, injected in batches into the apical third, and condensed vertically with a hand plugger to form apical plugs at the end of immature roots with and without periapical lesions [17]. Clinical indications for performing an apical plug include: (1) apex greater than 50–60 ISO in diameter, (2) immature apex, (3) irregular apical morphology, (4) canal morphology with parallel walls, (5) internal resorptions, (6) and orthograde root canal filling in case of subsequent apical surgery.

5.2 MTA Apical Plug Outcome

Since the introduction of MTA as an apical plug and an alternative to CH dressing, several studies have reported higher success and survival rates of the MTA apical plug compared with the conventional apexification technique using CH. In outcome assessment, success rates of CH ranged from 79 to 96% [10, 18], while higher healing rates (81–100%) were reported for MTA [19–21]. In direct comparisons between the two techniques, MTA resulted in less persistent disease [19]. Studies evaluating MTA success rates after a period of CH intracanal medication (1–6 weeks) showed a success rate of more than 90% in the median period (follow-up between 12 and 35 months) [22]. Sarris et al. reported a clinical success rate of 94.1% and a radiographic success rate of 76.5% at a mean follow-up of 12.5 ± 2.9 months in 17 nonvital permanent incisors treated with CH for at least one week followed by 3–4 mm MTA [23]. According to a systematic review and meta-analysis comparing the efficacy of CH and MTA for apexification of immature permanent teeth, which included only four studies (RCTs and observational studies), there was no difference in clinical and radiographic success rates or in the ratio of apical barrier formation between CH and MTA (clinical success rate: pooled odds ratio [OR] = 3.03, 95% CI: 0.42–21.72, $p = 0.271$; radiographic success rate: pooled OR = 4.30, 95% CI: 0.45–41.36, $p = 0.206$; apical barrier formation rate: pooled OR = 1.71, 95% CI: 0.59–4.96, $p = 0.322$). The actual difference between the two approaches is due to the time required for apical barrier formation, which is shorter for MTA than for CH (pooled difference in means = −3.58, 95% CI: from −4.91 to −2.25, $p < 0.001$) [24]. In a previous study, Chala et al. demonstrated that although similar results can be achieved with both techniques, the success rate of the MTA apical plug at final follow-up is 100%, while the success rate of apexification with CH reaches 92% [25]. Considering these two works, the choice of apexification techniques seems to depend only on the time needed to achieve clinical outcome and patient compliance. In the study by Pradhan et al., the total treatment time for MTA apical plug was 0.75 ± 0.5 months, whereas the time required to achieve a similar result with CH can be more than seven months (7 ± 2.5 months) [26]. Similar results were obtained in the study by Damle et al., which showed that the mean time for the apical barrier in the MTA group was 4.5 ± 1.6 months and for completion of the lamina dura was 4.1 ± 1.5 months, significantly shorter than in the CH group, which required 7.9 ± 2.5 and 6.4 ± 2.5 months, respectively ($p < 0.01$) [27]. In the retrospective study by Witherspoon et al., which analyzed the healing rate in a subgroup of 119 immature teeth treated with MTA apical plug in one (60.3% of the sample) or two appointments (39.7%), the percentage of healing was higher in the one-appointment group (96.5%) than in the two-appointment group (89%) [15]. In a recent systematic review comparing the success and survival rates of MTA apical plug and regenerative endodontic treatment (RET), the authors reported a pooled survival rate of 97.1% (95% CI: 93.7–100) and pooled success rates of 94.6% (95% CI, 90.2–99.1) for MTA apical plug and 97.8% (95% CI: 94.8–100) and 91.3% (95% CI, 84.5–98.2) for RET [28].

5.3 Other Apical Plug Materials

Although MTA is considered the gold standard for apical plug technique, it has several shortcomings such as long setting time (from 2 hours and 45 minutes to 4 hours), high cost, difficult handling, and the risk of post-treatment dyschromia, which is particularly detrimental in anterior teeth of young patients and because of the bismuth oxide added to MTA to improve radiopacity [29, 30]. For these reasons, and given the need for single-session treatment in patients requiring pharmacologic behavior management techniques such as sedation or anesthesia [31], bioceramics have been proposed as an alternative to MTA.

These materials have the same chemical and physical properties as MTA in terms of biocompatibility and for inducing the formation of a mineralized barrier. However, they offer additional advantages in terms of integration with the dentin component and replacement of bismuth oxide with zirconium oxide to improve the radiopacity of the material and ensure the chromatic stability of the elements for a better aesthetic outcome [32–34]. The main feature of these materials is bioactivity [35], the ability of the material to release calcium ions, electroconductivity, and the formation of a mineralized biological barrier between the cement and the dentin wall with deposition of HA [35–37]. Biodentine was introduced in 2010 as a calcium silicate-based bioactive cement with dentin-like mechanical properties and was formulated using MTA-based cement technology. It exhibits good sealing and mechanical properties with setting time of approximately 12 minutes. It can be used for a single visit apexification procedure, does not cause discoloration [38, 39], and has less radiopacity compared to MTA [40]. In a study conducted on 80 maxillary anterior teeth evaluating the apical microleakage of Biodentine compared to MTA in orthograde apical plugs and the effect of Biodentine thickness on sealability, Biodentine showed similar results to MTA in terms of microleakage and sealability without considering the thickness of the apical plug [41]. In a recent study, Abbas et al. showed that a 4-mm-thick Biodentine apical plug had the lowest bacterial leakage, followed by 2-mm MTA and 4-mm MTA, whereas a 2-mmthick Biodentine apical plug had the highest bacterial leakage [42]. However, the current literature is inconclusive regarding the efficacy of Biodentine when used as an apical plug. In a study, investigating the sealing ability of Biodentine with and without phosphate-buffered saline, Cechella et al. reported a lower sealing ability of Biodentine compared to MTA [43].

Positive results on the ability of Biodentine come from two recent randomized clinical trials. In the first study, Yadav et al. demonstrated apexification in 100% of teeth treated using Biodentine or MTA on a sample of 60 patients (age: 6–15 years). In the most recent randomized clinical trial [44], Tolibah et al. evaluated the radiographic and clinical outcomes of Biodentine apical plugs versus MTA in 30 immature roots of 24 permanent lower first molars with apical lesions. They showed no statistically significant differences in the periapical index scale between the two groups at 6- and 12-months after treatment, as well as the presence of an apical calcified barrier at 12 months in the Biodentine group [17]. In recent years, a calcium-enriched mixed cement (CEM cement), a hydrophilic tooth-colored cement that releases CH during and after setting, has been proposed as an apical plug that has similar sealing ability to MTA but offers some advantages over MTA because of its ability to set in an aqueous environment with a short setting time [45].

5.4 Apical Plug Technique

The apical plug technique aims to seal large and irregular apexes permanently. Achieving this goal is particularly complex given the anatomical variability of immature teeth, making it difficult to determine the working length [46, 47]. The MTA apical plug procedure is performed in two sessions.

5.4.1 In the First Session

A dressing with CH is applied after disinfection of the root canal system and before insertion of the MTA, to alter the low pH of the inflamed periapical tissue, which could affect adhesion and hardening of the MTA if not adequately controlled [48].

5.4.2 In the Second Session

After completion of irrigation, a 4-mm MTA apical plug is placed 1 mm from the radiographic apex using a carrier or plugger [49].

However, some clinicians prefer to place the MTA apical plug in a single session to take advantage of the production of CH during the mixing phase of the material itself and to reduce the risk of difficulty in removing CH during the second session, a difficulty that can lead to a defect in the seal if the material is resorbed over time.

MTA has a "wet sand" consistency and is difficult to handle when placed in the root canal. To overcome this disadvantage, some instruments have been proposed,

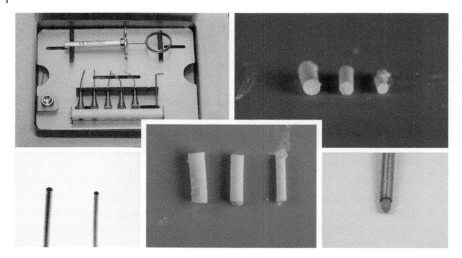

Figure 5.1 Map system – intro kit with 3NiTi tips. Blue 1.30 mm, red 1.10, yellow 0.90 mm.

of which the Micro Apical Placement System (MAP system) (Produits Dentaires SA, Switzerland) is the most used (Figure 5.1). The system consists of a tip with a plugger and a bayonet connection into which a plastic piston is inserted for the placement of the material, and a screw attachment with accessories that can be adapted to the clinical situation (see Online Video). The tips, often made of NiTi and available in three outer diameters of 0.90, 1.10, and 1.30 mm, can be bent into the desired shape and return to their original shape when heated.

After preparation, the MTA is loaded into the tip and extruded in the shape of a 4/5-mm cylinder. In 2013, Giovarruscio et al. proposed a new technique for filling root canals with an apical diameter greater than 0.4 mm. In this method, three Thermafil carriers (Maillefer, Switzerland) of increasing size are used as flexible pluggers starting 1, 2, and 3 mm short of the apex. This technique allows to check the consistency of the MTA during insertion to avoid a hard, shaped material that can lead to a short apical plug [50] and can be inserted in curved canals [51]. In addition, other accessories such as cones and microbrushes with a cylindrical shape are available to handle MTA directly in the canal.

After the MTA is placed, a cotton pellet, paper tip, or moistened brush head is placed over the MTA layer to supply the moisture needed to activate the material and thus for its hardening. After a few days, the MTA is checked with an endodontic instrument, and if it is not correctly hardening, the procedure is repeated; otherwise, the conventional obturation procedure can be continued. Table 5.1 showcases few of the procedural challenges faced with their predictable solutions. Solutions adopted in case of procedural challenges are shown in Figure 5.2.

Table 5.1 Problems and solutions.

Problem	Solution
Short apical plug or with gap and non-hardened material	1) Irrigate the canal with sterile water and make a hole through the material using a 20 k-File. 2) Hydrate the material, which will be enough to recompact it to the correct length.
Short apical plug with hardened material	Remove by ultrasound
Abundant extrusion of MTA beyond the apex	1) Irrigate over the apex with saline 2) Repeat the apical plug procedure
Material not hardened after 72 h	1) Remove the MTA 2) Check there is no spontaneous drainage from the canal 3) Repeat the apical plug procedure using the same or a different material

(a)   (b)   (c)

(d)

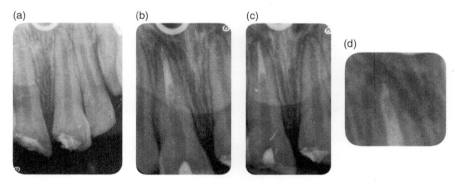

Figure 5.2 Long setting time – voids or short plug – (a) Preoperative radiography of the tooth 2.1 – pulp necrosis due to trauma, (b) Apical plug in MTA with evident voids in the periapical area, (c) Correction of the apical plug in the same session, (d) Detail of the vacuum in the periapical area.

5.4.3 Extra-Apical Resorbable Barriers

Overfilling is the major limitation of the apical plug technique. In immature roots, the proper placement of materials such as MTA or bioceramics depends on the apical diameter or the morphology and the path of the root canal walls, which may be parallel, convergent, or divergent depending on root development [10, 52–55]. Therefore, in immature permanent elements with periapical lesions, where there is a significant loss of coronal structure insufficient for adequate definitive restoration, and in those that are in stages 3 and 4 of root development, an alternative treatment to traditional apexification aimed at promoting continuous root development is recommended: the modified apexification technique (MAT) to prevent material extrusion.

Clinical Case 5.1

An asymptomatic 23-year-old patient presented with a discolored and nonviable element 1.1. Radiograph revealed apical radiolucency and incomplete root formation. After applying a resorbable fibrin matrix beyond the apex, a 4-mm MTA apical plug was placed in a single session. Unfortunately, the matrix was not very compact, and the MTA was extruded beyond the apex during apexification. Because the patient was asymptomatic in the months following treatment, it was decided to wait and monitor the patient with radiographic controls. After 10 years, the MTA was resorbed beyond the apex, while the material inside the root was stable and showed no changes (Figure 5.3).

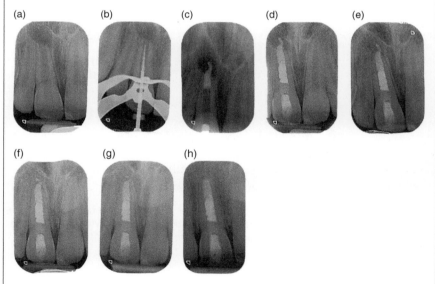

(a) (b) (c) (d) (e)

(f) (g) (h)

Figure 5.3 (a) Diagnosis. (b) Electronic WL. (c) MTA Apical plug. (d) One-year radiographic recall. (e) Two years radiographic recall. (f) Four years radiographic recall. (g) Six years radiographic recall. (h) 10 years radiographic recall.

Take to Home Message

1) The correct placement of a resorbable extra-apical barrier is essential to avoid extra-apical extrusions of MTA.
2) Even if the MTA is extruded beyond the apex, bone regeneration can occur.

In this technique, an absorbable collagen matrix [56, 57] or a platelet-rich fibrin matrix [58] is placed more than 1–2 mm from the root apex to create an artificial boundary that prevents the apical plug material from penetrating the periapical tissues, thereby reducing the risk of treatment failure [59]. In addition, a recent study reported that the placement of an extra-apical barrier allowed complete radiographic healing or resorption of the periapical lesion after a follow-up period of two years [60]. In this case, the MAP system can also be used with a metal plugger (Prexo by Deppeler) with two different diameters and resorbable fibrin positioned behind the apex to avoid uncontrolled extrusion of the material.

After positioning the rubber dam and adequately removing the bacterial biofilm from the root canal, a resorbable collagen matrix approximately 3 mm thick is placed in the canal approximately 1–2 mm from the apex to prevent extrusion of material into the periapical tissue. The apical plug of MTA (approximately 3 mm thick) is then placed over the collagen matrix. The canal space is subsequently filled with hot gutta-percha, and the access space is permanently restored. If the root canal has angles of different lengths, the apical sounding technique (AST) is recommended to place the matrix beyond the apex to follow the irregularity of the apex.

The use of modern electronic apex locators of generation III or IV, used as an aid in the operative phase, allows the clinician to precisely position the matrix when treating elements with irregular apexes and/or divergent root canal walls is required. This procedure is particularly favored by using a new experimental technique, the AST. This involves examining the root canal system circumferentially to understand its natural anatomy, including any irregularities and/or inclinations with respect to the long axis of the tooth, which are also obstacles to achieving an adequate seal. Using different endodontic files or manual pluggers to avoid errors during the transcription phase, the four main working lengths are identified: vestibular, palatal, mesial, and distal. The differences between the individual lengths are an expression of the inclination of the plane of the apical foramen in relation to the long axis of the tooth: the more inclined the foramen, the greater the difference between the measurements. The AST is, therefore, a new experimental and noninvasive technique that makes it possible to determine the exact positioning of the collagen barrier along the entire apical perimeter, thus achieving a perfect marginal seal by the restorative material without underfilling or overfilling (Figure 5.4).

5.4.4 Apical Sounding Technique Procedure

After drying and cleaning the root canal, the fibrin is introduced with a metal plugger connected to the apical detector by placing it on the walls of the root canal and bringing it to electronic working length so that the fibrin follows the anatomy or angle of the root canal and is placed just behind the apex. Next, MTA is loaded

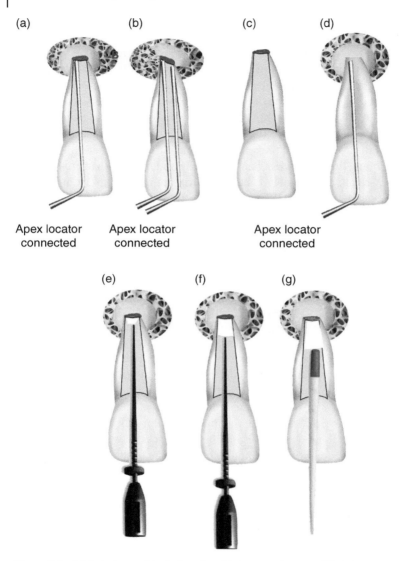

(a)   (b)   (c)   (d)

Apex locator   Apex locator   Apex locator
connected   connected   connected

(e)   (f)   (g)

Figure 5.4 (a) Apical sound technique in wide but regular apex. Fibrin is placed in front of Prexo plugger and pushed down until the apex locator signs "over." (b) In case of angle and wide and irregular apex, the WL can be variable; the reason why the fibrin is placed over the apex moving up and down the Prexo plugger keeping it connected to the apex locator. In this way, fibrin can be placed following the angle and material for the apical plug seal the entire area of the apex ideally without uncontrolled extrusions. (c) Wide apex. (d) Fibrin placed over the apex with press plugger connected to the apex locator. (e) MTA extrusion and first plug made with Thermafil carrier 1mm shorter than WL. (f) After one or two applications of MTA the plugger will remain automatically shorter than 4/5 mm. (g) Paper point with moisture placed inside canal for 72 hours for improving the MTA set.

into the MAP system extrusion, set in the canal, and compacted with the plastic plugger positioned 0.5 mm below the working length until the plastic plugger remains short compared to the working length of approximately 4 mm (Figure 5.4e). All material traces on the root canal walls are then cleaned with a moist paper cone or a moist micro brush (Figure 5.4g). If the procedure is completed in one session, the canal is filled with thermoplastic gutta-percha, while a wet paper cone is used in the case of a second session.

Clinical Case 5.2

A 54-year-old patient who had already been treated with a prosthetic crown after trauma and subsequent necrosis complained of pain. Radiographic examination revealed a periapical lesion and a fistula on tooth 1.1. Because the patient did not want to have an apicoectomy because of her dental anxiety and an apex of 0.80 mm was present, orthograde retreatment with direct MTA apexification and the subsequent composite filling was performed. After perforating the crown, and performing cleaning and shaping of the root canal, an apex locator with a metal plugger was used to monitor the proper apical placement of the resorbable matrix. The post-treatment radiograph shows the correct placement of the MTA without extrusion (Figures 5.5–5.7).

(a)   (b)

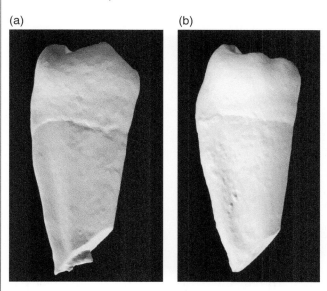

Figure 5.5 Microscopic vision of a large apex – in vitro test in apexes with an angle of 45°. Microscopic vision of the large apex. (a) Apical plug in MTA with extrusion in the point where the apex is shorter; (b) Apical sound technique without MTA extrusion because of the application of a matrix at 45°.

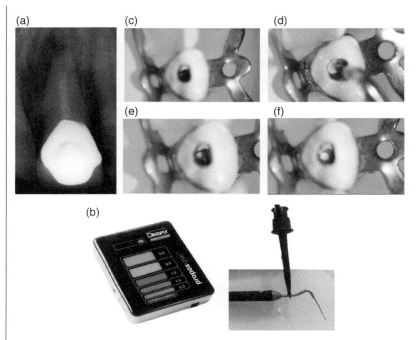

Figure 5.6 (a) Preoperative radiograph: Presence of a periapical lesion, a reabsorbed apex with a 45° angle and a prosthetic crown; (b) Attachment of an apex locator to the plugger for proper positioning of the extra apical fibrin or matrix. (c) Microscopic vision of the apex. (d) Fibrin insertion with the plugger connected to the apex locator. (e) Positioning of the extra apical fibrin. (f) Placement of the MTA apical plug.

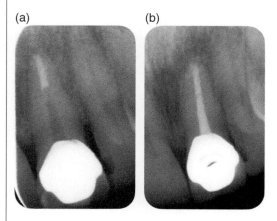

Figure 5.7 (a) Postoperative Rx showing the correct positioning of the MTA and the lack of extrusion. (b) Two-year radiographic recall.

Take to Home Message

1) Always use the apex locator attached to the plugger to place the extra apical fibrin.
2) If access is through a metal crown, ensure that the measurement is not disturbed.

In contrast to previous procedures which do not allow tissue regeneration, the modified apexification technique has shown continuous root development with a significant increase in length, thickened root canal walls, and a closed apex [60]. This different outcome is likely because of the length of the root, the size of the apical foramen, and the preservation of the progenitor cells. The modified apexification technique preserves a space of only 4–5 mm at the apical level, which is quickly filled by the granulation tissue if the foramen is large, without causing cell damage [60].

Another advantage of the modified apexification technique through AST compared to RET is the ability to make restoration with a post or composite resin in the canal space. The dual-flow composite and fiber posts placed only 3 mm deep significantly strengthen the root of the immature tooth and reduce the risk of fracture [61–63]. Furthermore, like regenerative procedures and in contrast to the conventional apical plug technique without an extra apical barrier, the modified apexification technique also aims to mature the root further and thus increase the corona-to-radicular ratio, which also seems to occur more frequently than in cases treated with RET [60].

5.5 Complex Clinical Cases

Clinical Case 5.3

A 36-year-old patient with a history of trauma complained of pain in nonvital teeth 11 and 12. Radiographic examination revealed a large periapical radiolucency. The diagnosis was pulpal necrosis. After drying the root canal, an MTA apical plug was placed in the root canals, followed by backfilling with gutta-percha and direct filling with composite (Figure 5.8).

(a) (b) (c) (d) (e)

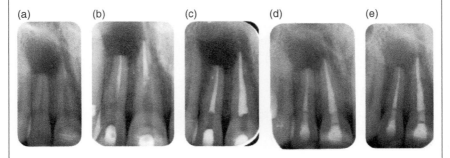

Figure 5.8 (a) Preoperative radiography. (b) MTA Apical plug – Teeth: 11 and 12. (c) Backfilling in gutta-percha. (d) Six months radiographic recall. (e) One-year radiographic recall. (f) Two years radiographic recall. (g) Three years radiographic recall. (h) Five years radiographic recall. (i) Seven years radiographic recall.

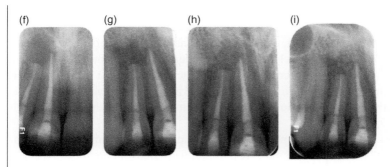

(f) (g) (h) (i)

Figure 5.8 (Continued)

Take to Home Message

1) For retreatments, an intraoperative radiograph should be taken before performing AP to ensure that there are no apical gutta-percha remnants that could compromise the quality of the seal.
2) If multiple treatments are performed with MTA, they should be done in the same session to better master the technique. Therefore, always plan sufficient time for all treatments.

Clinical Case 5.4

A 19-year-old male patient with previous trauma to nonvital tooth 21 required aesthetic treatment because of dyschromia. Radiographic examination revealed that the root was not formed, and the apex had an angle of 45°. Given the large apical diameter and root length, orthograde treatment with direct MTA apexification followed by aesthetic reconstruction with composite was planned (Figures 5.9–5.11).

Take to Home Message

1) For short canals, remember to always put the rubber stopper on the irrigation needle.
2) For short canals, use a microscope for direct observation, if possible.

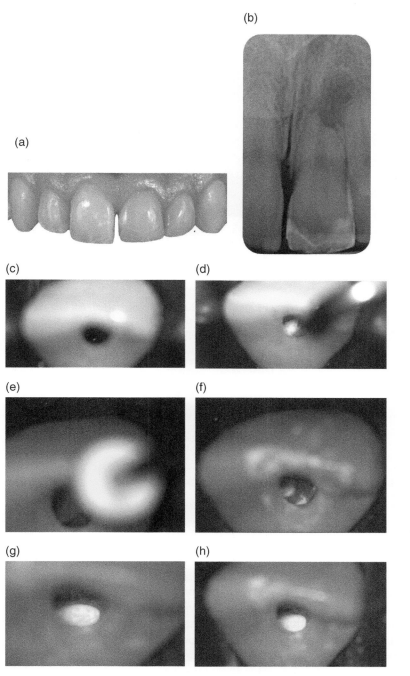

Figure 5.9 (a) Initial aesthetic condition. (b) Pretreatment radiography showing periapical lesion due to pulp necrosis and incomplete apical formation. (c) Operative microscope vision of the apex. (d) Positioning of the matrix by apical sound technique. (e) MTA positioning by MAP System. (f) MTA extruded by Map System. (g, h) MTA adapted apically.

(a)   (b)   (c)   (d)

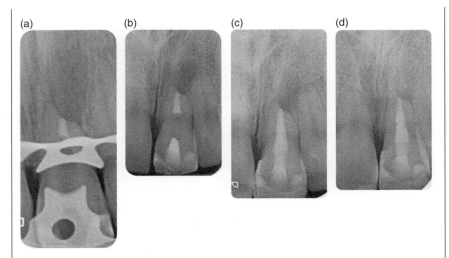

Figure 5.10   (a) Intraoperative Rx and apical plug. (b) Postoperative radiography. (c) Control at six months with direct restoration in composite. (d) Control at one year that showed the complete healing of the periapical lesion.

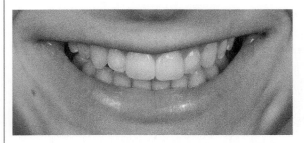

Figure 5.11   Direct composite restorations. *Source:* Courtesy of Dr. S. Bertoni.

Clinical Case 5.5

An asymptomatic 35-year-old patient complained of aesthetic problems related to element 11, and the history revealed that the element had been previously treated for trauma. After diagnostic testing and radiographic examination, which revealed a periapical granuloma, large apex, and coronal discoloration, pulpal necrosis and a periapical lesion were diagnosed. Orthograde treatment was performed with an MTA apical plug, a provisional post, and a prosthetic crown (Figures 5.12–5.15).

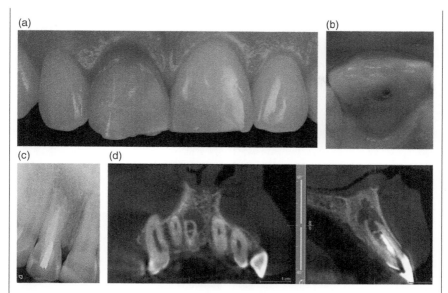

Figure 5.12 (a) Element 11 discoloration. (b) Metal pin. (c) Preoperative Rx showing difficulty of treatment and motivating therapeutic choice. (d) CBCT: diameter and irregularity of the apex.

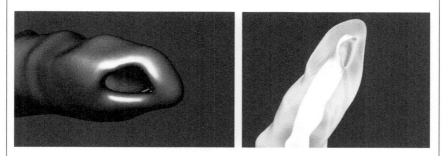

Figure 5.13 3D reconstruction of the periapical anatomy.

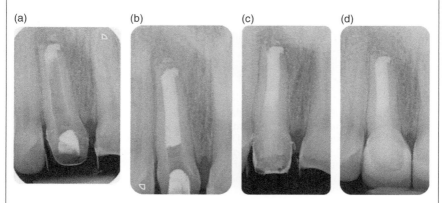

Figure 5.14 (a) Apical plug. (b) Gutta-percha backfilling. (c) Fiber post and provisional crown. (d) Final crown and three-year follow-up.

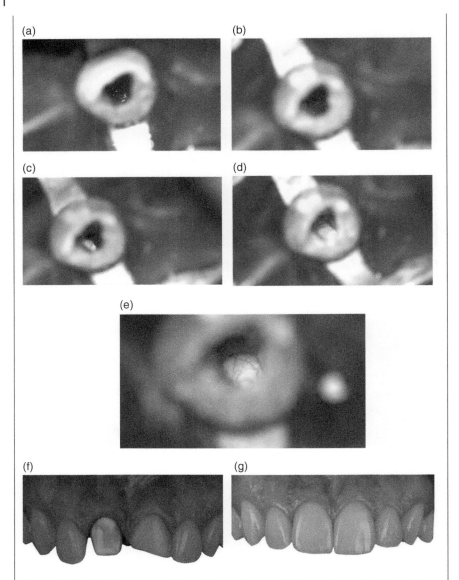

Figure 5.15 (a) Microscopic vision of the periapex with internal invagination of the periapical inflammatory tissue. (b) Apical microscopic vision after the positioning of the extra apical resorbable matrix. (c) MTA application. (d) First 2 mm of MTA. (e) 4-mm MTA control. (f) Initial aesthetic condition. (g) Aesthetic condition at three-year follow-up. *Source:* Courtesy of Dr. L. Tacchini.

> **Take to Home Message**
>
> 1) If the apex is irregular, the print and try technique is recommended to reduce the operator factor.
> 2) The alternative of apical surgery should always be considered and evaluated with the patient as it may be more conservative and decisive.

References

1 Araujo, P.R.S., Silva, L.B., Neto, A. et al. (2017). Pulp revascularization: a literature review. *The Open Dentistry Journal* 10: 48–56.

2 Seltzer, S. (1988). The root apex. In: *Endodontology: Biologic Considerations in Endodontic Procedures* (ed. S.K. Seltzer and P. Krasner), 1–30. Philadelphia: Lea& Febiger.

3 Torabinejad, M. (2014). *Mineral Trioxide Aggregate – Properties and Clinical Applications*. Oxford: Wiley Blackwell.

4 Cooper, P.R., Takahashi, Y., Graham, L.W. et al. (2010). Inflammation-regeneration interplay in the dentine-pulp complex. *Journal of Dentistry* 38 (9): 687–697.

5 Sheehy, E.C. and Roberts, G.J. (1997). Use of calcium hydroxide for apical barrier formation and healing in non-vital immature permanent teeth: a review. *British Dental Journal* 183 (7): 241–246.

6 Torabinejad, M., Hong, C.U., Lee, S.J. et al. (1995). Investigation of mineral trioxide aggregate for root-end filling in dogs. *Journal of Endodontia* 21 (12): 603–608.

7 Magura, M.E., Kafrawy, A.H., Brown, C.E. Jr., and Newton, C.W. (1991). Human saliva coronal microleakage in obturated root canals: an in vitro study. *Journal of Endodontia* 17 (7): 324–331.

8 Andreasen, J.O., Farik, B., and Munksgaard, E.C. (2002). Long-term calcium hydroxide as a root canal dressing may increase risk of root fracture. *Dental Traumatology* 18 (3): 134–137.

9 Andreasen, J.O., Munksgaard, E.C., and Bakland, L.K. (2006). Comparison of fracture resistance in root canals of immature sheep teeth after filling with calcium hydroxide or MTA. *Dental Traumatology* 22 (3): 154–156.

10 Cvek, M. (1992). Prognosis of luxated non-vital maxillary incisors treated with calcium hydroxide and filled with gutta-percha. A retrospective clinical study. *Endodontics & Dental Traumatology* 8 (2): 45–55.

11 Doyon, G.E., Dumsha, T., and von Fraunhofer, J.A. (2005). Fracture resistance of human root dentin exposed to intracanal calcium hydroxide. *Journal of Endodontia* 31 (12): 895–897.

12 Rosenberg, B., Murray, P.E., and Namerow, K. (2007). The effect of calcium hydroxide root filling on dentin fracture strength. *Dental Traumatology* 23 (1): 26–29.

13 Kobayashi, Y. and Shimizu, E. (2019). Current and future views on cell-homing-based strategies for regenerative endodontics. In: *Clinical Approaches in Endodontic Regeneration* (ed. H.F. Duncan and P.R. Cooper). Switzerland: Springer.

14 Shabahang, S., Torabinejad, M., Boyne, P.P. et al. (1999). A comparative study of root-end induction using osteogenic protein-1, calcium hydroxide, and mineral trioxide aggregate in dogs. *Journal of Endodontia* 25 (1): 1–5.

15 Witherspoon, D.E., Small, J.C., Regan, J.D., and Nunn, M. (2008). Retrospective analysis of open apex teeth obturated with mineral trioxide aggregate. *Journal of Endodontia* 34 (10): 1171–1176.

16 Bidar, M., Disfani, R., Gharagozloo, S. et al. (2010). Medication with calcium hydroxide improved marginal adaptation of mineral trioxide aggregate apical barrier. *Journal of Endodontia* 36 (10): 1679–1682.

17 Tolibah, Y.A., Kouchaji, C., Lazkani, T. et al. (2022). Comparison of MTA versus biodentine in apexification procedure for nonvital immature first permanent molars: a randomized clinical trial. *Children (Basel)*. 9 (3): 410.

18 Kerekes, K., Heide, S., and Jacobsen, I. (1980). Follow-up examination of endodontic treatment in traumatized juvenile incisors. *Journal of Endodontia* 6 (9): 744–748.

19 El-Meligy, O.A. and Avery, D.R. (2006). Comparison of apexification with mineral trioxide aggregate and calcium hydroxide. *Pediatric Dentistry* 28 (3): 248–253.

20 Pace, R., Giuliani, V., Pini Prato, L. et al. (2007). Apical plug technique using mineral trioxide aggregate: results from a case series. *International Endodontic Journal* 40 (6): 478–484.

21 Simon, S., Rilliard, F., Berdal, A., and Machtou, P. (2007). The use of mineral trioxide aggregate in one-visit apexification treatment: a prospective study. *International Endodontic Journal* 40 (3): 186–197.

22 Holden, D.T., Schwartz, S.A., Kirkpatrick, T.C., and Schindler, W.G. (2008). Clinical outcomes of artificial root-end barriers with mineral trioxide aggregate in teeth with immature apices. *Journal of Endodontia* 34 (7): 812–817.

23 Sarris, S., Tahmassebi, J.F., Duggal, M.S., and Cross, I.A. (2008). A clinical evaluation of mineral trioxide aggregate for root-end closure of non-vital immature permanent incisors in children-a pilot study. *Dental Traumatology* 24 (1): 79–85.

24 Lin, J.C., Lu, J.X., Zeng, Q. et al. (2016). Comparison of mineral trioxide aggregate and calcium hydroxide for apexification of immature permanent teeth: a systematic review and meta-analysis. *Journal of the Formosan Medical Association* 115 (7): 523–530.

25 Chala, S., Abouqal, R., and Rida, S. (2011). Apexification of immature teeth with calcium hydroxide or mineral trioxide aggregate: systematic review and meta-analysis. *Oral Surgery, Oral Medicine, Oral Pathology, Oral Radiology, and Endodontics* 112 (4): e36–e42.

26 Pradhan, D.P., Chawla, H.S., Gauba, K., and Goyal, A. (2006). Comparative evaluation of endodontic management of teeth with unformed apices with mineral trioxide aggregate and calcium hydroxide. *Journal of Dentistry for Children (Chicago, IL)* 73 (2): 79–85.

27 Damle, S.G., Bhattal, H., and Loomba, A. (2012). Apexification of anterior teeth: a comparative evaluation of mineral trioxide aggregate and calcium hydroxide paste. *The Journal of Clinical Pediatric Dentistry* 36 (3): 263–268.

28 Torabinejad, M., Nosrat, A., Verma, P., and Udochukwu, O. (2017). Regenerative endodontic treatment or mineral trioxide aggregate apical plug in teeth with necrotic pulps and open apices: a systematic review and meta-analysis. *Journal of Endodontia* 43 (11): 1806–1820.

29 Camilleri, J. (2020). Current classificarion of bioceramic materials in endodontics. In: *Bioceramic Materials in Clinical Endodontics* (ed. J. Camilleri). Cham, Switzerland: Springer.

30 Felman, D. and Parashos, P. (2013). Coronal tooth discoloration and white mineral trioxide aggregate. *Journal of Endodontia* 39 (4): 484–487.

31 Chung, S.H., Chun, K.A., Kim, H.Y. et al. (2019). Periapical healing in single-visit endodontics under general anesthesia in special needs patients. *Journal of Endodontia* 45 (2): 116–122.

32 Abuelniel, G.M., Duggal, M.S., and Kabel, N. (2020). A comparison of MTA and biodentine as medicaments for pulpotomy in traumatized anterior immature permanent teeth: a randomized clinical trial. *Dental Traumatology* 36 (4): 400–410.

33 Camilleri, J. (2015). Staining potential of neo MTA plus, MTA plus, and biodentine used for pulpotomy procedures. *Journal of Endodontia* 41 (7): 1139–1145.

34 Camilleri, J. (2013). Investigation of biodentine as dentine replacement material. *Journal of Dentistry* 41 (7): 600–610.

35 Parirokh, M. and Torabinejad, M. (2010). Mineral trioxide aggregate: a comprehensive literature review – part I: chemical, physical, and antibacterial properties. *Journal of Endodontia* 36 (1): 16–27.

36 Parirokh, M. and Torabinejad, M. (2010). Mineral trioxide aggregate: a comprehensive literature review – part III: clinical applications, drawbacks, and mechanism of action. *Journal of Endodontia* 36 (3): 400–413.

37 Parirokh, M. and Torabinejad, M. (2014). Calcium silicate-based cements. In: *Mineral Trioxide Aggregate, Properties and Clinical Application*, 1e (ed. M. Torabinejad), 284–320. Oxford, UK: Wiley Blackwell.

38 Bachoo, I.K., Seymour, D., and Brunton, P. (2013). A biocompatible and bioactive replacement for dentine: is this a reality? The properties and uses of a novel calcium-based cement. *British Dental Journal* 214 (2): E5.

39 Camilleri J. Biodentine™. (2022). The dentine in a capsule or more? https://www.septodontcorp.com/wp-content/uploads/2018/02/Biodentine-Article-0118-LOW.pdf (June 2022).

40 Kaur, M., Singh, H., Dhillon, J.S. et al. (2017). MTA versus Biodentine: review of literature with a comparative analysis. *Journal of Clinical and Diagnostic Research* 11 (8): ZG01–ZG05.

41 Bani, M., Sungurtekin-Ekci, E., and Odabas, M.E. (2015). Efficacy of Biodentine as an apical plug in nonvital permanent teeth with open apices: an in vitro study. *BioMed Research International* 2015: 359275.

42 Abbas, A., Kethineni, B., Puppala, R. et al. (2020). Efficacy of mineral trioxide aggregate and Biodentine as apical barriers in immature permanent teeth: a microbiological study. *International Journal of Clinical Pediatric Dentistry* 13 (6): 656–662.

43 Cechella, B., de Almeida, J., Kuntze, M., and Felippe, W. (2018). Analysis of sealing ability of endodontic cements apical plugs. *Journal of Clinical and Experimental Dentistry* 10 (2): e146–e150.

44 Yadav, A., Chak, R.K., and Khanna, R. (2020). Comparative evaluation of mineral trioxide aggregate, Biodentine, and calcium phosphate cement in single visit apexification procedure for nonvital immature permanent teeth: a randomized controlled trial. *International Journal of Clinical Pediatric Dentistry* 13 (Suppl 1): S1–S13.

45 Adel, M., Nima, M.M., Shivaie Kojoori, S. et al. (2012). Comparison of endodontic biomaterials as apical barriers in simulated open apices. *ISRN Dentistry* 2012: 359873.

46 Camp, J.H. (2008). Diagnosis dilemmas in vital pulp therapy: treatment for the toothache is changing, especially in young, immature teeth. *Journal of Endodontia* 34 (7 Suppl): S6–S12.

47 Hulsmann, M. and Pieper, K. (1989). Use of an electronic apex locator in the treatment of teeth with incomplete root formation. *Endodontics & Dental Traumatology* 5 (5): 238–241.

48 Lee, Y.L., Lee, B.S., Lin, F.H. et al. (2004). Effects of physiological environments on the hydration behavior of mineral trioxide aggregate. *Biomaterials* 25 (5): 787–793.

49 Yeung, P., Liewehr, F.R., and Moon, P.C. (2006). A quantitative comparison of the fill density of MTA produced by two placement techniques. *Journal of Endodontia* 32 (5): 456–459.

50 Giovarruscio, M., Uccioli, U., Malentacca, A. et al. (2013). A technique for placement of apical MTA plugs using modified Thermafil carriers for the filling of canals with wide apices. *International Endodontic Journal* 46 (1): 88–97.

51 Woelber, J.P., Bruder, M., Tennert, C., and Wrbas, K.T. (2014). Assessment of endodontic treatment of c-shaped root canals. *Swiss Dental Journal* 124 (1): 11–15.

52 Friend, L.A. (1966). The root treatment of teeth with open apices. *Proceedings of the Royal Society of Medicine* 59 (10): 1035–1036.

53 Friend, L.A. (1967). The treatment of immature teeth with non-vital pulps. *Journal of the British Endodontic Society* 1 (2): 28–33.

54 Kling, M., Cvek, M., and Mejare, I. (1986). Rate and predictability of pulp revascularization in therapeutically reimplanted permanent incisors. *Endodontics & Dental Traumatology* 2 (3): 83–89.

55 Moore, A., Howley, M.F., and O'Connell, A.C. (2011). Treatment of open apex teeth using two types of white mineral trioxide aggregate after initial dressing with calcium hydroxide in children. *Dental Traumatology* 27 (3): 166–173.

56 Sood, R., Kumar Hans, M., and Shetty, S. (2012). Apical barrier technique with mineral trioxide aggregate using internal matrix: a case report. *The Compendium of Continuing Education in Dentistry* 33 (6): e88–e90.

57 Vanka, A., Ravi, K.S., and Shashikiran, N.D. (2010). Apexification with MTA using internal matrix: report of 2 cases. *The Journal of Clinical Pediatric Dentistry* 34 (3): 197–200.

58 Yadav, P., Pruthi, P.J., Naval, R.R. et al. (2015). Novel use of platelet-rich fibrin matrix and MTA as an apical barrier in the management of a failed revascularization case. *Dental Traumatology* 31 (4): 328–331.

59 Khatavkar, R.A. and Hegde, V.S. (2010). Use of a matrix for apexification procedure with mineral trioxide aggregate. *Journal of Conservative Dentistry* 13 (1): 54–57.

60 Songtrakul, K., Azarpajouh, T., Malek, M. et al. (2020). Modified apexification procedure for immature permanent teeth with a necrotic pulp/apical periodontitis: a case series. *Journal of Endodontia* 46 (1): 116–123.

61 Katebzadeh, N., Dalton, B.C., and Trope, M. (1998). Strengthening immature teeth during and after apexification. *Journal of Endodontia* 24 (4): 256–259.

62 Ree, M.H. and Schwartz, R.S. (2017). Long-term success of nonvital, immature permanent incisors treated with a mineral trioxide aggregate plug and adhesive restorations: a case series from a private endodontic practice. *Journal of Endodontia* 43 (8): 1370–1377.

63 Seto, B., Chung, K.H., Johnson, J., and Paranjpe, A. (2013). Fracture resistance of simulated immature maxillary anterior teeth restored with fiber posts and composite to varying depths. *Dental Traumatology* 29 (5): 394–398.

6

Regeneration in Endodontics with Clinical Cases

Abhishek Parolia[1,2], Maya Feghali[3], and Catherine Ricci[4]

[1] *Department of Endodontics, University of Iowa College of Dentistry and Dental Clinics, Iowa City, IA, USA*
[2] *School of Dentistry, International Medical University, Kuala Lumpur, Malaysia*
[3] *Private Practice, Paris, France*
[4] *University of Nice-Sophia Antipolis, Nice, France*

CONTENTS

6.1 Introduction

Regenerative endodontics has been defined as "the biologically based procedures designed to replace damaged structures, including dentin, root structures, as well as cells of the pulp-dentin complex" [1]. Regenerative endodontics was introduced first by Nygaard-Ostby in 1961, then revised by Iwaya et al. in 2001 [2]. Since then, many studies have been published showing favorable outcomes in terms of radiographic healing of periapical tissues, thickening and lengthening of dentinal walls, and apical closure [3, 4].

The regenerative procedure has been shown to be an alternative approach to the established apexification procedures for the treatment of permanent immature necrotic teeth as a result of caries, trauma, or development anomalies. Various intracanal medicaments (ICMs) including calcium hydroxide have been used for the apexification procedure. However, calcium hydroxide is not advocated any more because of the long time needed to create an apical barrier, weakening its effect on the thin dentin walls and, thus, increasing the susceptibility of cervical root fracture [5].

Current treatment protocols recommend the placement of mineral trioxide aggregate (MTA) plug to close the apical foramen. Although MTA induces a mineralized barrier apically, this approach does not allow further root maturation.

The new way of regenerative thinking seems to be promoted by the limitations of the use of calcium hydroxide or MTA apexification that consist in creating a physical barrier against which the root canal filling can be achieved without any improvement in root dimensions, and susceptibility to root fractures because of thin canal walls and poor root-crown ratio [5].

Regenerative procedure based on the usage of stem cells, scaffold, and growth factors aims to repair and replace damaged tooth structures and restore normal pulp function in combination with regaining pulp connective tissue vitality in necrotic and infected teeth [6]. According to the American Association of Endodontics (AAE) [7], the degree of success of functional pulp regeneration is largely measured by parameters including elimination of symptoms and evidence of bony healing, increased root wall thickness and/or increased root length, and positive response to vitality testing for the tertiary goal ([7])

Different terms have been used to describe this procedure, such as regeneration, pulp revascularization, and revitalization. These techniques have been suggested to make use of the stem cells present at the apical area of immature teeth after induction of bleeding from the periapical tissue. The blood clot formation has been shown to allow repopulation of the root canal with vital tissues and promote continued deposition of hard tissue and further root development by the deposition of mineralized tissue [5].

This regenerative technique, commonly known as the regenerative endodontics procedure (REP), is based on the following prerequisites [5]:

1) Presence of stem cells
2) Complete disinfection of the root canals
3) Provision of a scaffold within a root canal
4) Provision of a signal to the stem cells so that they can differentiate

Stem cells of the apical papilla (SCAP) have been shown to play a major role in regeneration techniques. Stem cell population growth into the root canal system is achieved mainly through induction of bleeding from the periapical area. This has been supported by the work of Lovelace et al. [8] who showed a 400- to 600-fold increase in mesenchymal stem cell markers in blood collected from root canals in comparison to the levels found in systemic blood samples. Apical papilla cells differentiate into root primary odontoblasts and promote root dentin formation by continuing their normal physiological development after revascularization procedures [9]. Although the exact nature of the tissue repopulating the root canal system is still unclear, histological studies have reported fibroblasts, blood vessels, collagen, cementoblasts and osteoblasts, and pulp-like tissue in the repopulating tissue [9].

6.2 Factors Affecting the Clinical Outcome of REP

6.2.1 Etiology

The etiology or cause of the pulpal necrosis or apical periodontitis has shown to influence the outcome of REPs. Caries, trauma (30%), or development anomalies including dens evaginatus (22%) [10] have been the main causes of permanent immature teeth developing necrosis and apical periodontitis and, thereby, treated by REP [10].

REPs performed to treat cases with dens evaginatus have shown to have better prognosis than cases with trauma as a cause for the pulpal damage [10]. This could be explained by the fact that trauma to the tooth structure can lead to the induction of root resorption and cause damage to the Hertwig's epithelial root sheath and apical papilla, thus affecting the outcome of REP negatively [9].

The vast majority of failed REP cases were diagnosed with necrotic pulp and some form of apical pathosis. The presence of established periapical pathosis in cases of a necrotic pulp with an immature apex may render the disinfection of these cases more challenging and less predictable. Various studies have observed and demonstrated a relationship between the duration of pulp necrosis and the outcome of REP [11]. Similarly, Vishwanat et al. [12] found a significant association between the presence of periapical radiolucency and the lack of increased root wall thickness due to the residual bacterial biofilms modifying the osteogenic differentiation of stem cells from the apical papillae.

6.2.2 Type of the Tooth

The establishment of REPs constitutes an adequate treatment option for immature single-rooted necrotic teeth with apical periodontitis. However, there is little evidence for the complete acceptance of REP as a predictable and reproductible treatment option in posterior immature teeth with pulpal necrosis and apical periodontitis [13, 14].

In addition to the type of the tooth, the size of the apical foramen/opening has been considered a significant predictor factor for the success of REP. Better outcome is noted when the size of the apical foramen ranges between 0.5 and 1 mm [13].

6.2.3 Induction of Bleeding and Blood Clot

The evoked-bleeding step in REPs triggers the significant accumulation of undifferentiated stem cells into the root canal space as shown by [8], where these cells might contribute to the regeneration of pulpal tissues.

Once the blood clot is formed after the induction of bleeding, it acts as a physical scaffold for the three-dimensional organization of the newly formed tissue and releases necessary stem cell population growth factors for cell growth and cell differentiation [15].

Although the bleeding induction during REP is a critical step, the outcome of it remains unpredictable. Multiple cases have reported difficulties initiating bleeding even after the use of vasoconstrictor-free anesthetic solution[10, 11]. Furthermore, some studies, despite the lack of bleeding induction, have shown radiographic continuing of thickness of canal walls and apical closure [10, 16].

Digka et al. [17] did not observe any significant differences in the histological outcome with the success or failure to induce apical bleeding and a blood clot formation, and, in fact, concluded that the periapical tissues may be injured during the apical bleeding procedure with an endodontic file. Therefore, the bleeding induction step may not be a clear predictor to determine the outcome of REP.

6.2.4 Disinfection of the Root Canal System

Thorough disinfection of the root canal system plays a crucial role in the success of REPs. Various irrigants and ICMs have been attempted to achieve thorough disinfection.

Sodium hypochlorite (NaOCl) has been used with different concentrations as the only irrigation solution, or in combination with other irrigants for REPs. Despite the fact that this irrigant has been shown to have a potent antimicrobial action that dissolves organic matter at concentrations superior to 3%, it is probably cytotoxic to periodontal ligament cells and stem cells of apical papilla [5, 15]. For this reason, clinical considerations of the AAE recommend the use of lower concentrations of NaOCl in REPs [18].

In some publications, chlorhexidine (CHX) in addition to NaOCl has been used to disinfect the root canal system because of the antimicrobial activity and substantivity of CHX. The use of CHX and NaOCl should not be recommended because it leads to the formation of a cytotoxic orange precipitate named Para-Chloroaniline [19, 20]. Additionally, 2% CHX solution has been found to induce serious cytotoxic effects on stem cells, so clinicians should avoid using it as the final irrigant in REPs [15, 21].

The use of NaOCl solution followed by EDTA is now widely recommended [10]. It has been shown that EDTA promotes greater survival of the SCAPs and the release of trapped stem cells from the dentin [21]. In another study, [22] found that EDTA used for final irrigation partially countermands the effect of high concentrated NaOCl on the survival of stem cells. EDTA helps create a microenvironment in root canals that promotes the survival/proliferation and the differentiation of SCAPs, and has a positive impact on the outcome of REP [10, 22].

Various ICMs have been tried and tested in REPs, however, triple antibiotic paste (TAP) (100 mg metronidazole, 100 mg minocycline, and 100 mg ciprofloxacin) has been shown to have efficient bactericidal effect and potency to eradicate microorganisms from the infected dentin of root canals. Lately, the use of minocycline has been eliminated from the TAP to avoid potential tooth discoloration [23].

6.2.5 Coronal Barrier

A poor coronal seal can have a negative impact on the outcome of REPs. Achieving a good coronal seal is of utmost necessity in maintaining a sterile root canal environment, preventing future contamination and, thereby, failure of the procedure.

Nowadays, several materials such as MTA, Biodentine and bioceramic-based ready-to-use materials are gaining popularity in providing a coronal seal because of their advantages, including biocompatibility and tissue-conductive properties. Glass ionomer cements (GICs) or composite resin are placed above the MTA-based materials to ensure a hermetic seal [24, 25].

6.3 Materials used for REP

NaOCl at a concentration between 1 and 2.5% can be used as the main solution for irrigation. However, biocompatibility considerations should be considered to protect any vital remnants of SCAP.

In addition to NaOCl, EDTA has been found to offer advantages by increasing the survival ability of the stem cells and releasing growth factors trapped within the dentin matrix [13]. EDTA conditioning of the dentin promotes cell adhesion, migration, and differentiation toward the dentin [26]. Thus, EDTA irrigation as a final rinse before the induction of bleeding was likely to act favorably on the formation of new mineralized tissue [13, 26].

Various ICMs including calcium hydroxide and TAP have been used to disinfect the root canals in REPs with no differences observed in terms of treatment outcomes [27, 28].

Calcium hydroxide as an ICM has been historically used to induce the formation of a hard tissue barrier at the root apex because of its antimicrobial activity, high pH, or its direct effect on the periapical soft tissues [28, 29]. However, there are several limitations relating to its use, such as the long time required for hard tissue barrier formation, possibility of root canal contamination during the process, multiple, repeated dressings, and patient's compliance. Additionally, long-term application of calcium hydroxide may affect the dentinal structure and reduce the fracture resistance of teeth.

MTA has gained popularity amongst clinicians over the years. The principal components of MTA powder include tricalcium silicate, tricalcium aluminate, tricalcium oxide, and silicate oxide, and liquid can be distilled water or saline.

MTA has multiple benefits compared to calcium hydroxide as the apexification procedure can be completed in one or two visits with no dependence on the patient's compliance, and greatly reducing the risk of reinfection of the tooth and fracture [4]. It also possesses high radiopacity, less solubility, good antimicrobial property, and high biocompatibility, bioactivity, and regenerative potential. However, ProRoot MTA has some limitations as well, including high cost, long setting time (70–175 minutes) and difficulty handling.

Therefore, a few other alternatives such as Biodentine (Septodont, Saint-Maur-des-Fosses, France), and OrthoMTA (BioMTA, Seoul, Korea) can also be tried to manage these kinds of cases.

Biodentine contains tricalcium silicate as a core material and calcium chloride in liquid form. It has a few major advantages over MTA, including fast setting time (6–10 minutes), high compressive strength (100–300 MPa), and flexure strength (34 MPa). However, the radiopacity of Biodentine is lesser (3.5 mm of equivalent thickness of aluminum) than MTA (7 mm of equivalent thickness of aluminum). It also possesses less solubility, good antimicrobial property, and high biocompatibility, bioactivity, and regenerative potential similar to MTA [30, 31].

OrthoMTA, popularly known as grafting material, has similar composition to MTA with less heavy metal contents than MTA. It also possesses similar properties like MTA and Biodentine with a setting time of 180–360 minutes. It forms an interfacial hydroxyapatite layer between OrthoMTA and the root canal wall and prevents microleakage. It also creates intratubular mineralization and entombs the remaining microorganisms [32, 33].

6.4 Key Points to Remember While Performing REPs

- A permanent tooth with an open apex poses a different set of challenges compared to the tooth with a mature root apex.
- Incomplete root and thin dentinal walls make the tooth more susceptible to fracture, and compromised crown to root ratio may cause increased mobility.
- Owing to the presence of fracture-prone thin dentinal wall, disinfection of the root canal system relies solely on chemical disinfection using irrigants and ICM.
- Careful selection of irrigants/ICMs is imperative to ensure successful outcomes. Calcium hydroxide/TAP/2% chlorhexidine can be used as an intracanal medication. However, each ICM may have its limitations.
- Extrusion of instruments/irrigants/ICMs and obturating material can lead to inflammation of periapical tissues and delay the healing process.
- To prevent extrusion of irrigants into periapical tissue, irrigating system with a negative pressure system such as an EndoVac or GentleWave system is recommended. Close-ended, single side vented needle should be used if positive pressure technique is used while irrigating the canal in open apex cases.
- Careful working length determination through an apex locator and reconfirming it with the intraoral periapical radiograph (IOPA) is recommended in open apex cases.
- Although MTA has been the material of choice because of its biocompatibility, it takes a long setting time, and a waiting period of a few hours may be needed after the placement of MTA to achieve hard set mass. An alternative fast-setting Biodentine material can be used.
- A very specific disinfected environment must be created in the root canal space for revascularization of the pulp to take place. A combination of antibiotics – specifically ciprofloxacin, metronidazole, and minocycline – has been shown to properly kill common endodontic pathogens in the infected root canal. The blood clot can be created by instrumenting the tooth beyond apex to approximately 1–2 mm to permit bleeding into the root canal system.
- Multiple theories for the mechanism of revascularization have been proposed and discussed. Current protocol of REP suggested by the AAE presents with its own sets of limitations. Therefore, careful case selection is imperative in determining case success.

Clinical Case 6.1

Patient Information

- Age: nine-year-old
- Gender: Male

Tooth

- Identification: Maxillary left lateral incisor (Tooth 22)
- Dental history: The patient came with a concern of dull pain in his front tooth and gum area.
- Clinical examination findings: Tooth 22 was sound but tender on palpation and percussion. The tooth was non-mobile and showed negative response on pulp sensibility tests. No periodontal pocket was detected. A small enamel defect in the middle of the cingulum was noticed under the microscope.
- Preoperative radiological assessment: Tooth 22 was immature with open root apex and a periapical lesion (Figure 6.1a). A dens in dente in the coronal third of the tooth could also be observed.
- Diagnosis: Pulpal necrosis with symptomatic apical periodontitis.

Treatment Plan

- After considering the patient's age, history, medical status, and clinical and investigations findings, a regenerative endodontic procedure (REP) was planned with the removal of dens in dente.
- After obtaining the written consent from the parents, an access cavity was prepared using endo access burs (Dentsply Maillefer, Ballaigues, Switzerland) under a local anesthetic injection with 4% articaine hydrochloride with epinephrine 1 : 200 000 (Primacaine, Acteon, France) and rubber dam isolation, dens in dente was removed using a diamond bur. The working length was previously evaluated on the preoperative radiograph (IOPA).
- The root canal was negotiated and irrigated with 10 ml of 2.5% NaOCl solution using EndoVac® (Kerr Dental Products, France), the canal was dried aspirating with the EndoVac. Nonsetting calcium hydroxide (Voco GmbH Germany) was placed in the root canal using Lentulo spiral for three weeks to disinfect the root canal and access was restored using glass ionomer cement (Fuji II, GC Corporation, Tokyo, Japan) for three weeks to achieve disinfection.
- At the second appointment, 4% articaine hydrochloride without epinephrine (Primacaine, Acteon, France) anesthetic solution was administered. Access to the root canal was achieved after removing the previous GIC restoration under rubber dam isolation. The canal was irrigated with 10 ml of 2.5% NaOCl solution plus 10 ml of 17% EDTA solution (SmearClear) (Kerr Dental Products, France) using EndoVac. The canal was dried aspirating with

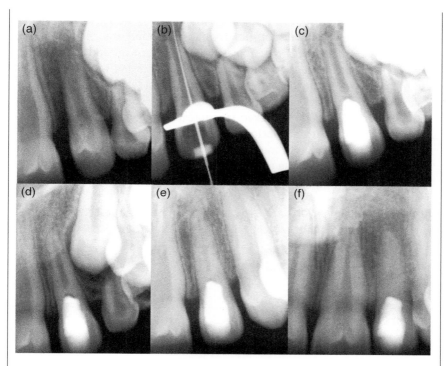

Figure 6.1 (a) Preoperative intra-oral radiograph showing immature tooth 22 with open root apex and a peri-apical lesion. (b) Inducing the bleeding by extending the file beyond the apex. (c) Placement of ProRoot MTA in the coronal third of the root as a part of REP. (d) Three months follow up showing satisfactory periapical healing and slight closure of root apex. (e, f) Eight years and 11 years follow up radiograph of tooth 22 showing complete closure of the root apex and resolution of peri-apical lesion.

    the EndoVac MicroCannula. Thereafter, a K file size 25 (Dentsply Maillefer, Ballaigues, Switzerland) was introduced into the canal beyond the apex to induce bleeding in the root canal space (Figure 6.1b).

- After achieving the bleeding, a blood clot was formed after almost 10 minutes. A piece of collagen membrane was placed on the blood clot to have a barrier on which the biomaterial could be placed. In this case, white ProRoot MTA (Dentsply International) powder mixed with sterile water in a 0.26 WP ratio was placed using MTA Gun System (Dentsply Sirona, Ballaigues, Switzerland) and the access cavity was restored with GIC Fuji II (GC Corporation, Tokyo, Japan) (Figure 6.1c).
- The patient was recalled for follow-up after one month to assess the clinical signs and symptoms, such as absence of tenderness to percussion or

palpation, swelling, locally deep periodontal probing defect, tooth mobility, and condition of coronal seal. An intraoral radiograph was taken to assess the reduction/absence of periapical lesion. The clinical and radiographic findings of the three months' follow-up visits suggested satisfactory healing process with a small barrier into the root canal just apically to the collagen membrane and narrowing of the root canal space (Figure 6.1d). The GIC (Fuji II, GC Corporation, Tokyo, Japan) restoration was partially removed and a composite resin (Ivoclar Vivadent, Liechtenstein) restoration was done. The follow-up was done at regular intervals up to 11 years (Figure 6.1e and f) to ensure a positive outcome of the treatment.

Technical Aspects
In this case, calcium hydroxide was used as an ICM to disinfect the root canal. However, use of TAP or other ICM can be another alternative.

Clinical Case 6.2

Patient Information
- Age: eight-year-old
- Gender: Male

Tooth
Dental history: The patient came with a concern of pain in his front tooth. He gives a history of fractured teeth 11 and 21 after a traumatic injury, and broke the mesial angle of the right central incisor (tooth 11) and the incisal edge of the left central incisor (tooth 21). He got them restored six months ago.

- Clinical examination findings: Tooth 21 was tender on palpation and percussion with no mobility and periodontal pocket. It showed negative response on pulp sensibility tests.
- Preoperative radiological assessment: Coronal radiopacity suggesting composite resin restoration was observed approaching the pulp tissue. The root canal walls were parallel with no apical closure and a small periapical lesion (Figure 6.2a).
- Diagnosis: Pulpal necrosis with symptomatic apical periodontitis.

Treatment Plan
- After considering the patient's age, history, medical status, and clinical and investigations findings, two treatment options – revascularization or

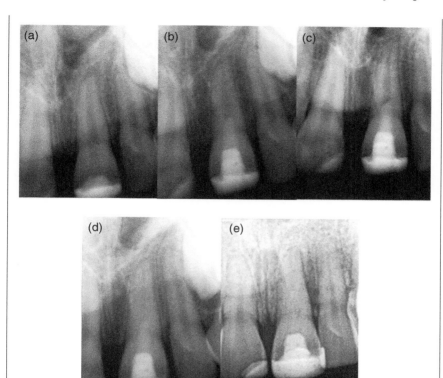

Figure 6.2 (a) Preoperative intraoral radiograph showing tooth 21 with open root apex and a periapical lesion; (b) Placement of Biodentine in the coronal third of the root as a part of REP; (c) Three months' follow-up showing satisfactory periapical healing and closure of root apex; (d, e) Five and eight years' follow up radiograph of tooth 21 showing complete closure of the root apex and resolution of periapical lesion.

apexification – were given to the parents. Possible outcomes were discussed, and parents decided to try revascularization.

- After obtaining the written consent from the parents, an access cavity was prepared using endo access burs (Dentsply Maillefer, Ballaigues, Switzerland) under a local anesthetic injection with 4% articaine hydrochloride with epinephrine 1 : 200 000 (Primacaine, Acteon, France) and rubber dam isolation. The working length was previously evaluated on the preoperative IOPA.
- The root canal was negotiated and irrigated with 20 ml of 2.5% NaOCl solution plus 10 ml of 17% EDTA solution (SmearClear) (Kerr Dental Products, France) using EndoVac® (Kerr Dental Products, France), the canal was dried aspirating with the EndoVac. In this appointment, non-setting calcium

hydroxide (Voco GmbH, Germany), an ICM was placed into the root canal using a Lentulo spiral for three weeks to achieve disinfection and access was restored using GIC (Fuji II, GC Corporation, Tokyo, Japan).

- At the second appointment, 4% articaine hydrochloride without epinephrine (Primacaine, Acteon, France) anesthetic solution was administered. Access to the root canal was achieved after removing the previous GIC restoration under rubber dam isolation. The canal was irrigated with 20 ml of 17% EDTA solution (SmearClear) (Kerr Dental Products, France) using EndoVac. The canal was dried aspirating with the EndoVac MacroCannula. Thereafter, a K file size 25 (Dentsply Maillefer, Ballaigues, Switzerland) was introduced into the canal beyond the apex to induce bleeding in the root canal space.
- After achieving the bleeding, a blood clot was formed after almost 10 minutes. A piece of collagen membrane was placed on the blood clot to prevent the material from sinking into the root canal. In this case, Biodentine (Septodont, France) was placed on the collagen membrane and the access cavity was restored with GIC (Fuji II, GC Corporation, Tokyo, Japan) (Figure 6.2b).
- The patient was recalled for follow-up after one month to assess the clinical signs/symptoms and periapical status The clinical and radiographic findings of the three follow-up visits suggested satisfactory healing process with the tooth showing positive response to cold test, and the root canal started to close apically and laterally (Figure 6.2c). The follow-up was done at regular interval up to eight years (Figure 6.2d and e) to ensure a positive outcome of the treatment.

Technical Aspects
In this case, calcium hydroxide was used as ICM to disinfect the root canal. This shows that the thorough disinfection of the root canal space and forming a good quality blood clot may increase the success of revascularization procedure.

References

1 Murray, P.E., Garcia-Godoy, F., and Hargreaves, K.M. (2007). Regenerative endodontics: a review of current status and a call for action. *Journal of Endodontics* 33 (4): 377–390. https://doi.org/10.1016/j.joen.2006.09.013.
2 Iwaya, S., Ikawa, M., and Kubota, M. (2001). Revascularization of an immature permanent tooth with apical periodontitis and sinus tract. *Dental Traumatology* 17 (4): 185–187. https://doi.org/10.1034/j.1600-9657.2001.017004185.x.
3 Hargreaves, K.M., Diogenes, A., and Teixeira, F.B. (2013). Treatment options: biological basis of regenerative endodontic procedures. *Journal of Endodontics* 39 (3 supp): https://doi.org/10.1016/j.joen.2012.11.025.

4 Torabinejad, M., Nosrat, A., Verma, P., and Udochukwu, O. (2017). Regenerative endodontic treatment or mineral trioxide aggregate apical plug in teeth with necrotic pulps and open apices: a systematic review and meta-analysis. *Journal of Endodontics* 43 (11): 1806–1820. https://doi.org/10.1016/j.joen.2017.06.029.

5 Duggal, M., Tong, H.J., Al-Ansary, M. et al. (2017). Interventions for the endodontic management of non-vital traumatised immature permanent anterior teeth in children and adolescents: a systematic review of the evidence and guidelines of the European Academy of Paediatric Dentistry. *European Archives of Paediatric Dentistry: Official Journal of the European Academy of Paediatric Dentistry* 18 (3): 139–151. https://doi.org/10.1007/s40368-017-0289-5.

6 Langer, R., Vacanti, J.P., Vacanti, C.A. et al. (1995). Tissue engineering: biomedical applications. *Tissue Engineering* 1 (2): 151–161. https://doi.org/10.1089/ten.1995.1.151.

7 American Association of Endodontists (AAE) (2016). *Clinical Considerations for a Regenerative Procedure.* Chicago, IL, USA: American Association of Endodontists.

8 Lovelace, T.W., Henry, M.A., Hargreaves, K.M., and Diogenes, A. (2011). Evaluation of the delivery of mesenchymal stem cells into the root canal space of necrotic immature teeth after clinical regenerative endodontic procedure. *Journal of Endodontics* 37 (2): 133–138. https://doi.org/10.1016/j.joen.2010.10.009.

9 Lin, J., Zeng, Q., Wei, X. et al. (2017). Regenerative endodontics versus apexification in immature permanent teeth with apical periodontitis: a prospective randomized controlled study. *Journal of Endodontics* 43 (11): 1821–1827. https://doi.org/10.1016/j.joen.2017.06.023.

10 Almutairi, W., Yassen, G.H., Aminoshariae, A. et al. (2019). Regenerative endodontics: a systematic analysis of the failed cases. *Journal of Endodontics* 45 (5): 567–577. https://doi.org/10.1016/j.joen.2019.02.004.

11 Nosrat, A., Homayounfar, N., and Oloomi, K. (2012). Drawbacks and unfavorable outcomes of regenerative endodontic treatments of necrotic immature teeth: a literature review and report of a case. *Journal of Endodontics* 38 (10): 1428–1434. https://doi.org/10.1016/j.joen.2012.06.025.

12 Vishwanat, L., Duong, R., Takimoto, K. et al. (2017). Effect of bacterial biofilm on the osteogenic differentiation of stem cells of apical papilla. *Journal of Endodontics* 43 (6): 916–922. https://doi.org/10.1016/j.joen.2017.01.023.

13 Glynis, A., Foschi, F., Kefalou, I. et al. (2021). Regenerative endodontic procedures for the treatment of necrotic mature teeth with Apical Periodontitis: a systematic review and meta-analysis of randomized controlled trials. *Journal of Endodontics* 47 (Issue 6): 873–882. https://doi.org/10.1016/j.joen.2021.03.015.

14 Tzanetakis, G.N., Giannakoulas, D.G., Papanakou, S. et al. (2021). Regenerative endodontic therapy of immature permanent molars with pulp necrosis: a cases series and a literature review. *European Archives of Paediatric Dentistry* 22 (3): 515–525. https://doi.org/10.1007/s40368-020-00550-w.

15 Kontakiotis, E.G., Filippatos, C.G., Tzanetakis, G.N., and Agrafioti, A. (2015). Regenerative endodontic therapy: a data analysis of clinical protocols. *Journal of Endodontics* 41 (Issue 2): 146–154. https://doi.org/10.1016/j.joen.2014.08.003.

16 Yassen, G.H., Chu, T.M.G., Eckert, G., and Platt, J.A. (2013). Effect of medicaments used in endodontic regeneration technique on the chemical structure of human immature radicular dentin: an in vitro study. *Journal of Endodontics* 39 (2): 273. https://doi.org/10.1016/j.joen.2012.09.020.

17 Digka, A., Sakka, D., and Lyroudia, K. (2020). Histological assessment of human regenerative endodontic procedures (REP) of immature permanent teeth with necrotic pulp/apical periodontitis: a systematic review. *Australian Endodontic Journal* 46 (1): 140–153. https://doi.org/10.1111/aej.12371.

18 American Association of Endodontics (2013). Clinical considerations for regenerative procedures. www.aae.org/regenerativeendo/ (accessed 31 July 2013).

19 Cintra, L.T.A., Watanabe, S., Samuel, R.O. et al. (2014). The use of NaOCl in combination with CHX produces cytotoxic product. *Clinical Oral Investigations* 18 (3): 935–940. https://doi.org/10.1007/s00784-013-1049-5.

20 Orhan, E.O., Irmak, Ö., Hür, D. et al. (2016). Does para-chloroaniline really form after mixing sodium hypochlorite and chlorhexidine? *Journal of Endodontics* 42 (3): 455–459. https://doi.org/10.1016/j.joen.2015.12.024.

21 Trevino, E.G., Patwardhan, A.N., Henry, M.A. et al. (2011). Effect of irrigants on the survival of human stem cells of the apical papilla in a platelet-rich plasma scaffold in human root tips. *Journal of Endodontics* 37 (8): 1109–1115. https://doi.org/10.1016/j.joen.2011.05.013.

22 Martin, D.E., De Almeida, J.F.A., Henry, M.A. et al. (2014). Concentration-dependent effect of sodium hypochlorite on stem cells of apical papilla survival and differentiation. *Journal of Endodontics* 40 (1): 51–55. https://doi.org/10.1016/j.joen.2013.07.026.

23 Lin, L.M. and Rosenberg, P.A. (2011). Repair and regeneration in endodontics. *International Endodontic Journal* 44 (10): 889–906. https://doi.org/10.1111/j.1365-2591.2011.01915.x.

24 Alghamdi, F. and Alsulaimani, M. (2021). Regenerative endodontic treatment: a systematic review of successful clinical cases. *Dental and Medical Problems* 58 (4): 555–567. https://doi.org/10.17219/dmp/132181.

25 Peng, C., Yang, Y., Zhao, Y. et al. (2017). Long-term treatment outcomes in immature permanent teeth by revascularisation using MTA and GIC as canal-sealing materials: a retrospective study. *International Journal of Paediatric Dentistry* 27 (6): 454–462. https://doi.org/10.1111/ipd.12282.

26 Galler, K.M., Widbiller, M., Buchalla, W. et al. (2016). EDTA conditioning of dentine promotes adhesion, migration and differentiation of dental pulp stem cells. *International Endodontic Journal* 49 (6): 581–590. https://doi.org/10.1111/iej.12492.

27 Alfadda, S., Alquria, T., Karaismailoglu, E. et al. (2021). Antibacterial effect and bioactivity of innovative and currently used intracanal medicaments in regenerative endodontics. *Journal of Endodontics* 47 (8): 1294–1300. https://doi.org/10.1016/j.joen.2021.05.005.

28 Ruparel, N.B., Teixeira, F.B., Ferraz, C.C.R., and Diogenes, A. (2012). Direct effect of intracanal medicaments on survival of stem cells of the apical papilla. *Journal of Endodontics* 38 (10): 1372–1375. https://doi.org/10.1016/j.joen.2012.06.018.

29 Athanassiadis, B., Abbott, P.V., and Walsh, L.J. (2007). The use of calcium hydroxide, antibiotics and biocides as antimicrobial medicaments in endodontics. *Australian Dental Journal* 52: S64–S82. https://doi.org/10.1111/j.1834-7819.2007.tb00527.x.

30 Kaur, M., Singh, H., Dhillon, J.S. et al. (2017). MTA versus Biodentine: review of literature with a comparative analysis. *Journal of Clinical and Diagnostic Research: JCDR* 11 (8): ZG01–ZG05. https://doi.org/10.7860/JCDR/2017/25840.10374.

31 Malkondu, Ö., Karapinar Kazandağ, M.K., and Kazazoğlu, E. (2014). A review on biodentine, a contemporary dentine replacement and repair material. *BioMed Research International* 2014: 160951. https://doi.org/10.1155/2014/160951.

32 Lee, B.N., Son, H.J., Noh, H.J. et al. (2012). Cytotoxicity of newly developed ortho MTA root-end filling materials. *Journal of Endodontics* 38 (12): 1627–1630.

33 Yoo, J.S., Chang, S.W., Oh, S.R. et al. (2014). Bacterial entombment by intratubular mineralization following orthograde mineral trioxide aggregate obturation: a scanning electron microscopy study. *International Journal of Oral Science* 6 (4): 227–232. https://doi.org/10.1038/ijos.2014.30.

7

Management of Deep Caries with Bioceramics

Antonis Chaniotis[1] and Viresh Chopra[2,3,4]

[1] *Private Practice Endodontics, NKUA (National Kapodistrian University of Athens), Zografou, Greece*
[2] *Adult Restorative Dentistry, Oman Dental College, Muscat, Oman*
[3] *Endodontology, Oman Dental College, Muscat, Oman*
[4] *Bart's London School of Medicine and Dentistry, Queen Mary University, London, UK*

CONTENTS

7.1 Introduction

Enamel, dentin, and cementum protect the pulp from the oral environment [1]. An intact dental pulp could provide several defense mechanisms, possibly preventing bacterial invasion; hence, it is valuable to sustain an exposed pulp rather than meticulously replacing it with a synthetic root filling material [2]. Vital pulp therapy aims to preserve and maintain pulpal health in teeth where pulp has become infected and there are chances to reverse the health of the pulp for good [3]. Various treatment options for pulp-exposed teeth are direct pulp capping (DPC), pulpotomy, and pulpectomy. DPC is defined as "placing a dental material such as calcium hydroxide or mineral trioxide aggregate (MTA) directly on a mechanical or traumatic vital pulp exposure, thereby sealing the pulpal wound to facilitate the formation of reparative dentin and maintenance of the vital pulp" [4].

Historically, lack of success with DPC procedures was due to inefficient protocols and lack of materials that could generate a favorable environment that could lead to hard tissue formation [5, 6]. With the introduction of calcium silicate cements (MTA and bioceramics) and advanced treatment protocols, the DPC procedures have become more predictable with much favorable outcomes in comparison to the 30–85% success outcome of earlier times [7–9].

The aim of this case report is to present a case with management of infected pulp due to deep caries using the latest DPC protocols and recently introduced calcium silicate cements.

7.2   Patient Information

- Age: eight-year-old
- Gender: Female
- Medical history: Noncontributory

7.2.1   Tooth

- Identification: 36
- Dental history (include chief complaint): Pain in cold stimulus that lasts long after the stimulus
- Clinical examination findings: Leaking occlusal composite restoration
- Preoperative radiological assessment: Deep carious lesion and open apices (Figure 7.1a)
- Diagnosis (pulpal and periapical): Pulpal diagnosis consistent with irreversible pulpitis. Periapical diagnosis was normal periapical tissues.

7.3   Treatment Plan

- Preliminary procedures: Mandibular block infiltration anesthesia with 3% mepivacaine (Septodont, France). Rubber dam isolation and disinfection of the operating field with 2% chlorexidine (CHX) scrub. The carious lesion was removed with a diamond bur and the pulp roof was completely removed. Extensive bleeding was noticed that couldn't be controlled with pressure (Figure 7.1b).
- Treatment plan: The coronal pulp tissue was considered irreversibly inflamed and a decision was made to remove the inflamed pulp tissue up to the level that adequate hemostasis could be achieved. The aim was to preserve the apical pulp vital so that the apices of the tooth could be formed.

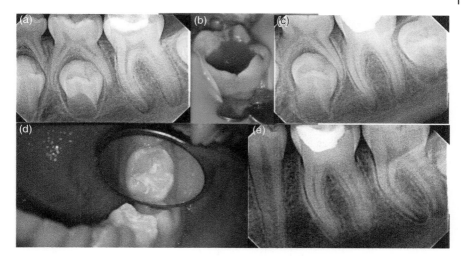

Figure 7.1 (a–e): Pictorial presentation of the DPC protocol followed to manage the pulp exposure due to deep carious lesion in a permanent tooth.

- Endodontic procedure: The pulp chamber was irrigated with 5% NaOCl solution. A sterile long-shafted round bur (Munce bur) was used to remove the pulp tissue remnants from the pulp chamber and the pulp tissue was removed to the level of the canal orifices. A sterile cotton pellet was soaked in 5% NaOCl solution and pressed against the canal orifices for five minutes. The cotton pellet was removed and hemostasis was achieved in the mesial canals but not in the distal canal. A smaller round bur was used to remove the pulp tissue deeper inside the distal canal orifice. The pulp resection site was rinsed with sterile water and another cotton pellet soaked in 5% NaOCl was pressed against the radicular pulp tissue.
- Canal preparation and obturation: After hemostasis was achieved, Biodentine (Septodont) material was prepared according to the manufacturer's instructions and placed over the pulp tissue to fill the whole pulp chamber. The material was delivered with an amalgam carrier and adapted with a microbrush. The material was allowed to set for 15 minutes and the tooth was restored with a composite resin restoration (Figure 7.1d). A postoperative radiograph was taken to be used as baseline (Figure 7.1c).
- Follow up: The patient missed all the scheduled follow-ups and returned four years later for evaluation. The four-year follow-up radiograph revealed normal periapical tissues and fully formed apices (Figure 7.1e). The tooth was asymptomatic and periodontal probing was within normal limits.

7.4 Learning Objectives

- Irreversibly inflamed pulp tissue might be predictably healed with deep pulpotomy procedures.
- The level of pulp resection is defined by the level at which effective pressure hemostasis can be achieved.
- Asepsis control is mandatory.

References

1 Yu, C. and Abbott, P.V. (2007). An overview of the dental pulp: its functions and responses to injury. *Australian Dental Journal* 52: S4–S6.

2 Barthel, C.R., Rosenkranz, B., Leuenberg, A., and Roulet, J.-F. (2000). Pulp capping of carious exposures: treatment outcome after 5 and 10 years: a retrospective study. *Journal of Endodontics* 26 (9): 525–528.

3 Hilton, T.J. (2009). Keys to clinical success with pulp capping: a review of the literature. *Operative Dentistry* 34 (5): 615–625.

4 Endodontists, A. (2003). *Glossary of Endodontic Terms*. Chicago: American Association of Endodontists.

5 Al-Hiyasat, A.S., Barrieshi-Nusair, K.M., and Al-Omari, M.A. (2006). The radiographic outcomes of direct pulp-capping procedures performed by dental students: a retrospective study. *The Journal of the American Dental Association* 137 (12): 1699–1705.

6 Linu, S., Lekshmi, M., Varunkumar, V., and Joseph, V.S. (2017). Treatment outcome following direct pulp capping using bioceramic materials in mature permanent teeth with carious exposure: a pilot retrospective study. *Journal of Endodontics* 43 (10): 1635–1639.

7 Baume, L.J. and Holz, J. (1981). Long term clinical assessment of direct pulp capping. *International Dental Journal* 31 (4): 251–260.

8 Auschill, T.M., Arweiler, N.B., Hellwig, E. et al. (2003). Success rate of direct pulp capping with calcium hydroxide. *Schweizer Monatsschrift für Zahnmedizin= Revue mensuelle suisse d'odonto-stomatologie= Rivista mensile svizzera di odontologia e stomatologia* 113 (9): 946–952.

9 Matsuo, T., Nakanishi, T., Shimizu, H., and Ebisu, S. (1996). A clinical study of direct pulp capping applied to carious-exposed pulps. *Journal of Endodontics* 22 (10): 551–556.

8

Regenerative Management of an Infected Pulp of a Permanent Tooth Using Bioceramics

Antonis Chaniotis[1] and Viresh Chopra[2,3,4]

[1] *Private Practice Endodontics, NKUA (National Kapodistrian University of Athens), Zografou, Greece*
[2] *Adult Restorative Dentistry, Oman Dental College, Muscat, Oman*
[3] *Endodontology, Oman Dental College, Muscat, Oman*
[4] *Bart's London School of Medicine and Dentistry, Queen Mary University, London, UK*

CONTENTS

8.1 Introduction

Newer advancements are happening in the field of endodontics on a daily basis. There have been significant advancements in regard to endodontic materials [1]. Bioceramics are amongst the recently introduced materials in endodontics and have changed the face of endodontics. They are biocompatible ceramic materials or metal oxides with enhanced physicochemical and biological properties that are useful in medicine and dentistry. They include alumina and zirconia, bioactive glass, glass ceramics, calcium silicates, hydroxyapatite and resorbable calcium phosphates, and radiotherapy glasses [2].

In endodontics they are used in obturation, perforation repair, retrograde filling, pulpotomy, resorption, apexification, and regenerative endodontics [3]. At present they are one of the best bioactive materials present in endodontics.

This case report aims to present the use of bioceramics as a regenerative material. It also emphasizes the protocol used for regeneration and disinfection in cases with longstanding infection.

8.2 Patient Information

- Age: nine-year-old
- Gender: Male
- Medical history: Noncontributory

8.2.1 Tooth

- **Identification:** Mandibular left first molar (tooth 36)
- **Dental history:** Intraoral swelling in the lower left mandibular area associated with a badly decayed first mandibular molar. Initial swelling had been managed with intraoral antibiotics regimen for one week before the visit to the clinic. The antibiotics regimen was amoxicillin 1 g twice per day for six days.
- **Clinical examination findings:** Distal decay and badly broken-down dental structures of tooth 36. Periodontal probing within normal limits. Asymptomatic. Negative thermal and electrical vitality testing for tooth 36.
- **Preoperative radiological assessment:** The preoperative intraoral periapical radiograph revealed a decayed first left mandibular molar with periapical lesion. The apices of tooth 36 were immature (Figure 8.1a, b).
- **Diagnosis (pulpal and periapical):** Pulpal diagnosis was pulp necrosis. Periapical diagnosis was chronic apical abscess.

8.3 Treatment Plan

Treatment alternatives included long-term root canal treatment using calcium hydroxide as intracanal medicament, MTA plug technique, or regenerative endodontics procedures. After presenting all treatment alternatives to the patient's guardian, a decision was made to attempt regenerative endodontic procedures. An informed consent was obtained.

The following regenerative endodontic procedure protocol was employed:

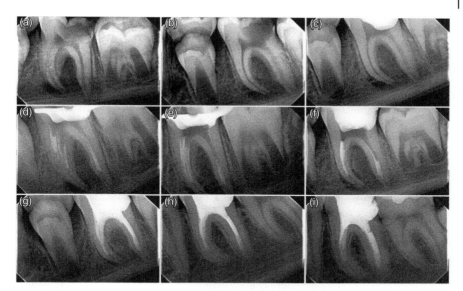

Figure 8.1 (a, b) Preoperative intraoral periapical radiograph. (c) Radiograpgh with intermediate antibiotic dressing. (d–f) Procedural MTA placement radiographs. (g) Postoperative radiograph. (h, i) Six-year follow-up radiographs from two different angulations.

8.3.1 First Visit

- The patient was anesthetized by using buccal infiltration anesthesia without vasoconstrictors (3% Mepivastesin, 3M ESPE).
- The rubber dam was placed. The operation field was disinfected by using 2% chlorhexidine scrub.
- The carious lesion was removed, the pulp cavity was accessed with a sterile diamond bur (Endo-Access Bur, Dentsply, Maillefer, Switzerland) and the contaminated content of the pulp chamber was rinsed away with copious 1.5% NaOCl irrigation through a slotted-end needle.
- The working length was estimated with a periapical radiograph along with apex locator and the canals were instrumented to a size of 45/04.
- The instrumented canals were rinsed with 10 ml of 1.5% NaOCl solution through a 27 G slotted-end needle fitted 2 mm short of working length.
- The canals were dried with capillary suction fitted 2 mm short of working length.
- A double antibiotic mixture powder containing equal parts of ciprofloxacin and metronidazole had been prepared by the compound pharmacy. The powder had been kept in the refrigerator. Just before use, the powder was mixed with sterile water to a slurry consistency (approximately 1000 mg/ml solution

is needed to create a pasty slurry consistency) and placed inside the instrumented canals with a lentullo spiral rotating 2 mm short of working length (Figure 8.1c).

- Glass ionomer was used as temporary coronal restorative material (Fuji IX GP).
- The patient was rescheduled after two weeks.

On clinical examination at the second visit, the tooth was asymptomatic and the temporary restoration in place.

8.3.2   Second Visit

- Anesthesia and rubber dam isolation were performed as in the first visit.
- The temporary restoration was removed with a sterile diamond bur and the double antibiotic mix was rinsed away with copious sterile saline irrigation through a slotted-end needle.
- The root canals were rinsed with 20 ml of 1.5% NaOCl solution through a 27 G slotted-end needle fitted 2 mm short of working length.
- The canals were dried with capillary suction fitted 2 mm short of working length.
- The EndoVac macro-cannula was fitted 2 mm short of working length and negative pressure irrigation with 10 ml of 1.5% NaOCl was performed in each canal.
- The canals were flooded with 1.5% NaOCl and left inside the canals non-agitated for 30 minutes.
- The canals were dried with capillary suction from the NaOCl solution and were flooded with 17% ethylenediaminetetraacetic acid (EDTA) through an EndoVac macro-cannula fitted in working length.
- The EDTA 17% was left for 10 minutes and then rinsed away with sterile water.
- The canals were dried with capillary suction fitted 2 mm short of working length.
- Bleeding was induced by mechanical irritation of the periapical tissues and rotational movement of a sterile apically pre-curved size 35 K-file.
- The apical third of the canals was allowed to fill with blood and we waited for 15 minutes for a clot to be formed.
- An MTA barrier of 4 mm thickness (MTA Angelus, Londrina, Brazil) was placed over each blood clot with an MTA applicator.
- The MTA material was adapted over the blood clot with a microbrush and a dry sterile cotton pellet (Figure 8.1d–f).
- MTA material was protected with injectable gutta-percha and the MTA remnants were removed with a grit blast of sodium bicarbonate sandblasting.

- The access cavity was rinsed with water and the tooth was restored with composite resin restoration (Figure 8.1g).
- A postoperative radiograph was taken to be used as baseline for future evaluations (Figure 8.1g).

8.3.3 Recall

The patient never returned for the scheduled follow up appointments. Six years later, the patient returned for the treatment of another tooth. Two follow-up radiographs with different angulation were taken for tooth 36 (Figure 8.1h, i). The six-year follow-up clinical evaluation revealed asymptomatic tooth with healthy soft tissues. The radiographic examination revealed complete periapical healing, continuous root development, dentinal wall thickening, and apical closure. No response to electric vitality testing was recorded.

8.4 Learning Objectives

The following key points should be beneficial to the clinician:

- Regenerative protocol to be used where indicated.
- Conventional disinfection measures may be insufficient in longstanding infections, therefore, advance technological methods should be used along with bioactive materials.
- Isolation of the tooth should be maintained in every visit to prevent it from contamination from saliva, blood, and other pathogenic microbiota.
- Recall of the patient is a must in every clinical treatment. This will help the clinician to authenticate their own protocol and help them in recording maintenance.
- The solid regenerative protocol suggested here might be predictable and reproducible in all cases of resistant intracanal infections.

References

1 Raghavendra, S.S., Jadhav, G.R., Gathani, K.M., and Kotadia, P. (2017). Bioceramics in endodontics – a review. *Journal of Istanbul University Faculty of Dentistry* 51 (3 Suppl 1): S128.
2 Nasseh, A. (2009). The rise of bioceramics. *Endodontic Practice* 2: 17–22.
3 Prati, C. and Gandolfi, M.G. (2015). Calcium silicate bioactive cements: biological perspectives and clinical applications. *Dental Materials* 31 (4): 351–370.

9

Endodontic Management of a Necrosed Pulp with Wide Open Apex

Antonis Chaniotis[1] and Viresh Chopra[2,3,4]

[1] *Private Practice Endodontics, NKUA (National Kapodistrian University of Athens), Zografou, Greece*
[2] *Adult Restorative Dentistry, Oman Dental College, Muscat, Oman*
[3] *Endodontology, Oman Dental College, Muscat, Oman*
[4] *Bart's London School of Medicine and Dentistry, Queen Mary University, London, UK*

CONTENTS

9.1 Introduction

Endodontic materials in clinical use face several challenges [1]. Ideally, these materials should be easy to use, visible in the radiograph, biocompatible, bioactive, have antimicrobial activity, be resorbable in tissues but resist resorption within tooth structures, be nonstaining to tooth structures, strengthen the tooth, be dimensionally stable, provide a permanent, high-quality seal with dental hard tissues yet be easy to replace, and have the mechanical strength that is optimal for the site and task they are used for [2].

Interestingly, regenerative approaches in endodontics have gained a lot of attention in the recent past. Preservation of vital and necrotic teeth with open apexes is

Bioceramics in Endodontics, First Edition. Edited by Viresh Chopra.
© 2024 John Wiley & Sons, Inc. Published 2024 by John Wiley & Sons, Inc.
Companion website: www.wiley.com/go/chopra/bioceramicsinendodontics

gaining popularity with the advent of calcium silicate materials [3–5]. Bioceramic cements are used as a material of choice in such treatments for a specific purpose. They are used as a mid-root or coronal plug after disinfection of the canal with an antibiotic paste. A blood clot is created in the apical canal or the canal is filled with platelet-rich plasma and the area is sealed coronally with bioceramic cement, which provides a permanent, high-quality seal [3]. A matrix such as CollaCote is often used apical to the cement to allow depth control for the cement. Materials with equal physicochemical and biological properties should be given priority. However, they should not stain the tooth structure [6].

The aim of this case report is to outline the detailed protocol to be used for regeneration using bioceramics with special emphases on the importance of recall to keep a track record of the case.

9.2 Patient Information

- Age: 16-year-old
- Gender: Female
- Medical history: Noncontributory

9.2.1 Tooth

- **Identification:** 11 (tooth 11)
- **Dental history:** Pain to percussion
- **Clinical examination findings:** At the time of the appointment, tooth 11 was percussion painful. Periodontal probing was within normal limits. Thermal and electrical vitality tests were negative.
- **Preoperative radiological assessment:** Radiographic examination revealed immature tooth 8 associated with a large periapical lesion (Figure 9.1a).
- **Diagnosis (pulpal and periapical):** Pulpal diagnosis was pulpal necrosis. Periapical diagnosis was symptomatic apical periodontitis.

9.3 Treatment Plan

Preliminary procedures: A decision was made to attempt calcium hydroxide apexification procedure. After administrating buccal infiltration anesthesia, the rubber dam was placed and stabilized with Wedjets (Coltene). The tooth was accessed with a diamond bur and purulent drainage was noticed. The wide canal was rinsed with sterile water followed by positive syringe irrigation of 6% NaOCl solution (CanalPro Extra, Coltene). The working length was estimated with a working length radiograph of an ISO 80 K-file fitted in place (Figure 9.1b).

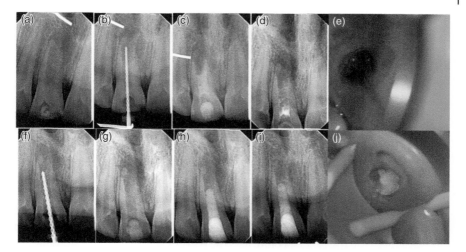

Figure 9.1 (a–j) Pictorial presentation of the protocol used for regeneration starting from preoperative until achieving a coronal seal.

Circumferential filling was done with the ISO 80 K-file and the canal was flooded with NaOCl 6%. The irrigation solution was activated with a 30 ultrasonic K-file (U-file, Mani, Japan) (3×20 seconds). The wide canal was dried, dressed with calcium hydroxide paste (UltraCal, Ultradent) and a temporary restoration of glass ionomer cement was placed (Figure 9.1c). The patient missed all the scheduled appointments and returned one year later with a big swelling and pain on percussion. A radiographic examination revealed the remnants of the calcium hydroxide dressing and a growing periapical lesion (Figure 9.1d). The tooth was accessed again, disinfected with 6% NaOCl, dressed with calcium hydroxide (UltraCal, Ultradent) and temporized with glass ionomer cement. Six months later, the patient returned to the dental clinic with pain on percussion.

- Treatment plan for the management of the endodontic mishap due to patient missing the appointments: A decision was made to try and deal with the persistent infection by using regenerative endodontic procedures.

9.4 Technical Aspects

The following regenerative protocol was used:

9.4.1 First Visit

- The patient was anesthetized by using buccal infiltration anesthesia with non-vasoconstriction containing anesthetic solution (3% Mepivastesin, 3M™ ESPE™).

- The rubber dam was placed and stabilized with Wedjets (Coltene). The operation field was disinfected by using 2% chlorhexidine scrub.
- The temporary restoration was removed with a diamond bur and the calcium hydroxide was rinsed away with sterile water irrigation (water for injection) through a slotted-end needle. Sterile water was used in large amounts to mechanically create a current and rinse the content of the wide canal away.
- The working length was verified again with a working length radiograph (Figure 9.1f).
- The wide canal was rinsed with 10 ml of 6% NaOCl solution through a 27 G slotted-end needle fitted 2 mm short of working length.
- The canal was dried with capillary suction fitted 2 mm short of working length.
- A double antibiotic mixture powder containing equal parts of ciprofloxacin and metronidazole had been prepared by the compound pharmacy. The powder had been kept in the fridge. Just before use, the powder was mixed with sterile water to a pasty slurry consistency (approximately 1000 mg/ml solution is needed to create a pasty slurry consistency) and placed inside the canal with a lentullo spiral rotating 2 mm short of working length.
- The tooth was temporized with glass ionomer restorative material (Fuji IX GP) and a radiograph was taken as baseline (Figure 9.1g).
- The patient was rescheduled after two weeks.

Two weeks later the tooth was asymptomatic.

9.4.2 Second Visit

- The patient was anesthetized by using buccal infiltration anesthesia with non-vasoconstriction containing anesthetic solution (3% Mepivastesin, 3M ESPE).
- The rubber dam was placed and stabilized with Wedjets. The operation field was disinfected by using 2% chlorhexidine scrub (Consepsis, Ultradent).
- The temporary restoration was removed with a diamond bur and the double antibiotics mix was rinsed away with sterile water irrigation (water for injection) through a slotted-end needle. Sterile water was used in large amounts to mechanically create a current and rinse the antibiotic content of the wide canal away.
- The wide canal was rinsed with 20 ml of 6% NaOCl solution through a 27 G slotted-end needle fitted 2 mm short of working length.
- The canal was dried with capillary suction fitted 2 mm short of working length.

- The EndoVac macro-cannula was fitted 1 mm short of working length and negative pressure irrigation with 10 ml of 6% NaOCl was performed.
- The canal was bubble-free flooded with 6% NaOCl and left inside the canal nonagitated for 30 minutes.
- The canal was dried with capillary suction from the NaOCl solution and was bubble-free flooded with 17% ethylenediaminetetraacetic acid (EDTA) through an EndoVac macro-cannula fitted in working length.
- The EDTA 17% was left for two minutes and then rinsed with sterile water.
- The canal was dried with capillary suction fitted 2 mm short of working length.
- Bleeding was induced by mechanical irritation of the periapical tissues and rotational movement of a sterile apically precurved size 40 K-file that was previously dipped in EDTA 17% solution.
- The canal was allowed to fill with blood until 2 mm below the gingival margin and we waited for 15 minutes for a clot to be formed (Figure 9.1e).
- Four shots (3 mm thick) of MTA Angelus white powder (Angelus, Londrina, Brazil) were placed over the blood clot with an MTA applicator (Angelus, Londrina, Brazil).
- The MTA powder was condensed over the blood clot with a micro-brush and adapted with a moist sterile cotton pellet (Figure 9.1j).
- The coronal MTA plug was protected with injectable gutta-percha plug and the cavity walls were cleaned and refreshed with a grit blast with aluminum oxide.
- The gutta-percha plug was removed with a DG-16 endodontic explorer and the tooth was restored with composite resin restoration (Figure 9.1h).

The two-year follow-up clinical and radiographic evaluation revealed an asymptomatic tooth with resolution of the periapical pathosis and apical closure (Figure 9.1i).

9.5 Learning Objectives

In the present paper, the use of a solid regenerative protocol able to shift the outcome of failing treatments is suggested. In longstanding infections, conventional disinfection measures might be insufficient to achieve infection control compatible with tissue healing, apical repair, and ingrowth of a viable tissue inside the empty canal space. The solid regenerative protocol suggested here might be predictable and reproducible in all cases of resistant intracanal infections.

References

1 Haapasalo, M., Parhar, M., Huang, X. et al. (2015). Clinical use of bioceramic materials. *Endodontic Topics* 32 (1): 97–117.

2 Ørstavik, D. (2005). Materials used for root canal obturation: technical, biological and clinical testing. *Endodontic Topics* 12 (1): 25–38.

3 Diogenes, A., Henry, M.A., Teixeira, F.B., and Hargreaves, K.M. (2013). An update on clinical regenerative endodontics. *Endodontic Topics* 28 (1): 2–23.

4 Sachdeva, G., Sachdeva, L., Goel, M., and Bala, S. (2015). Regenerative endodontic treatment of an immature tooth with a necrotic pulp and apical periodontitis using platelet-rich plasma (PRP) and mineral trioxide aggregate (MTA): a case report. *International Endodontic Journal* 48 (9): 902–910.

5 Jung, J.Y., Woo, S.M., Lee, B.N. et al. (2015). Effect of biodentine and bioaggregate on odontoblastic differentiation via mitogen-activated protein kinase pathway in human dental pulp cells. *International Endodontic Journal* 48 (2): 177–184.

6 Reyes-Carmona, J.F., Felippe, M.S., and Felippe, W.T. (2009). Biomineralization ability and interaction of mineral trioxide aggregate and white portland cement with dentin in a phosphate-containing fluid. *Journal of Endodontics* 35 (5): 731–736.

10

Clinical Application of Bioceramics as Direct Pulp Capping Material

Antonis Chaniotis[1] and Viresh Chopra[2,3,4]

[1] *Private Practice Endodontics, NKUA (National Kapodistrian University of Athens), Zografou, Greece*
[2] *Adult Restorative Dentistry, Oman Dental College, Muscat, Oman*
[3] *Endodontology, Oman Dental College, Muscat, Oman*
[4] *Bart's London School of Medicine and Dentistry, Queen Mary University, London, UK*

CONTENTS

10.1   Introduction

Bioceramic-based materials have a long history of use in tissue regeneration and medicine [1]. They were introduced to dentistry, specifically endodontics, as root and perforation repair materials or sealers [2–4]. Bioceramics consist of nanosphere particles, with the maximum dimension not exceeding $1 \times 10^{-3}\,\mu m$ [2], and mainly composed of tricalcium silicate, dicalcium silicate, calcium phosphate monobasic, amorphous silicon dioxide, and tantalum pentoxide [5]. Owing to their ability to penetrate dentinal tubules and to interact with dentine moisture, an optimum dimensional stability, and the least amount of shrinkage can be expected. When compared to white MTA, bioceramics have the advantage of being aluminum-free and inclusion of tantalum pentoxide as an opacifier [6].

Historically, Ca(OH)$_2$ medicament has been used for partial pulpotomy of the necrotic immature permanent tooth [7]. Bioceramics with an alkaline pH of 12.8 demonstrating effective antibacterial activity are becoming popular for the same clinical use [4].

The present clinical case report aims to present a similar case where bioceramic material has been used to manage a deep carious lesion leading to exposure of the pulp.

10.2 Patient Information

- Age: 9-year-old
- Gender: Male
- Medical history: Noncontributory

10.2.1 Tooth

- Identification: Mandibular left first molar (tooth 36)
- Dental history: Food impaction, extensive decay, referred for root canal treatment of tooth 36 (include chief complaint and the endodontic error with which the patient reported to your practice)
- Clinical examination findings: Mesial decay of tooth 36, asymptomatic
- Preoperative radiological assessment: Extensive carious lesion in approximation with the mesial pupal horn of tooth 36 (Figure 10.1a)
- Diagnosis (pulpal and periapical): Pulpal diagnosis consistent with reversible pulpitis. Periapical diagnosis consistent with normal periapical tissues.

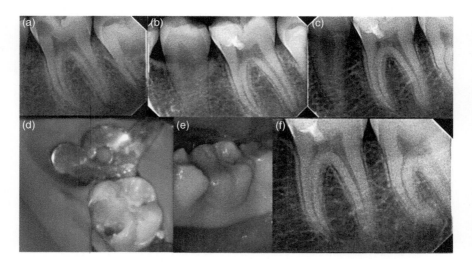

Figure 10.1 (a–f): Pictorial presentation of management of deep carious lesion using white MTA cement.

10.3 Treatment Plan

- Preliminary procedures: A mandibular block anesthesia was administered with 3% Mepivastesin (Septodont, France). The tooth was isolated with rubber dam and the operation field was disinfected with 2% chlorhexidine (CHX) scrub. The whole procedure was done under the magnification provided by a Global G6 operation microscope.
- Treatment plan for the management of the case: The mesio-occlusal carious lesion was removed with a high-speed round diamond bur together with the unsupported enamel. A new sterile low-speed round bur was used to remove the deepest parts of the carious lesion near the mesial pulp horn. Stepwise caries excavation was done with a hand instrument in proximity with the mesial pulp horn. A sterile cotton pellet was soaked with 2% CHX and was pressed against the cavity for surface disinfection before entering the mesial pulp horn.
- Stepwise root canal treatment procedure: A decision was made to perform partial pulpotomy of the partially infected young vital pulp. The carious lesion seemed clinically to be in proximity with the mesial pulp horn. A thin layer of carious dentine was separating the cavity from the mesial pulp horn. The operation field was rinsed with 2% CHX and a new sterile long-shafted bur was used to expose the pulp tissue (Figure 10.1d). The round bur was inserted 3 mm inside the pulp tissue to remove the infected parts of the pulp at the side of the pulp exposure. The debris created around the pulp exposure was rinsed away with sterile water irrigation. A sterile cotton pellet was soaked with 5% sodium hypochlorite solution and pressed against the bleeding area of the pulp exposure and inside the mesial pulp horn. The cotton pellet was left there for 10 minutes.
- Canal preparation (cleaning and disinfection procedure): The cotton pellet was removed and the pulp exposure was rinsed with sterile water irrigation. The excess moisture around the pulp exposure was dried with a sterile cotton pellet.
- Obturation (material and technique): MTA Angelus white material was mixed and prepared according to the manufacturer's instructions and the material was delivered over the pulp exposure with an amalgam carrier. The material was adapted in place with an inverted sterile ISO 80 paper point and protected with a shot of GI cement (Fuji). The cavity was restored with composite resin restoration in the same appointment (Figure 10.1e). A postoperative radiograph was taken to be used as baseline for the follow ups (Figure 10.1b).
- Additional information: The patient was recalled two weeks later for evaluation of pulp vitality. The pulp tissue responded well in cold sensitivity testing. The tooth was asymptomatic.
- The three- and five-year follow-up periapical radiographs revealed normal periapical tissues (Figure 10.1c, f). Periodontal probing was within normal limits and the tooth was asymptomatic. The pulp tissue responded well in cold sensitivity testing. A hard tissue bridging was evident in the periapical radiographs in contact with the MTA material. No sign of pulp tissue calcifications was noticed (Figure 10.1c, f).

10.4 Technical Aspects

Partial pulpotomy technique might predictably preserve the vitality of the pulp tissue. The most important parameter of the technique is to maintain strict asepsis control throughout the whole procedure. The operation field needs to be isolated and disinfected throughout the whole procedure. The excavation burs have to be replaced immediately after the removal of the infected carious lesion with new sterile ones before going to the deepest layers of the cavity. The area of the pulpotomy is disinfected with 5% NaOCl by distance irrigation and hemostasis is achieved with pressure. A bioactive plug is adapted over the resected pulp tissue and the tooth is restored in the same appointment. Previous MTA formulas had extended setting times and they had to be protected by GI cement before restoration. New bioceramic cements are fast setting and composite resin restoration can be achieved immediately without the need for an intermediate protective material.

10.5 Learning Objectives

- Partial pulpotomy is a predictable treatment approach when the pulp tissue is considered partially inflamed.
- Strict asepsis control is mandatory in vital pulp treatment procedures.

References

1 Marcacci, M., Kon, E., Moukhachev, V. et al. (2007). Stem cells associated with macroporous bioceramics for long bone repair: 6-to 7-year outcome of a pilot clinical study. *Tissue Engineering* 13 (5): 947–955.

2 De-Deus, G., Canabarro, A., Alves, G. et al. (2009). Optimal cytocompatibility of a bioceramic nanoparticulate cement in primary human mesenchymal cells. *Journal of Endodontics* 35 (10): 1387–1390.

3 Yuan, Z., Peng, B., Jiang, H. et al. (2010). Effect of bioaggregate on mineral-associated gene expression in osteoblast cells. *Journal of Endodontics* 36 (7): 1145–1148.

4 Damas, B.A., Wheater, M.A., Bringas, J.S., and Hoen, M.M. (2011). Cytotoxicity comparison of mineral trioxide aggregates and EndoSequence bioceramic root repair materials. *Journal of Endodontics* 37 (3): 372–375.

5 Chavez De Paz, L., Dahlén, G., Molander, A. et al. (2003). Bacteria recovered from teeth with apical periodontitis after antimicrobial endodontic treatment. *International Endodontic Journal* 36 (7): 500–508.

6 Park, J.-W., Hong, S.-H., Kim, J.-H. et al. (2010). X-Ray diffraction analysis of white ProRoot MTA and Diadent BioAggregate. *Oral Surgery, Oral Medicine, Oral Pathology, Oral Radiology, and Endodontology* 109 (1): 155–158.

7 Frank, A.L. (1966). Therapy for the divergent pulpless tooth by continued apical formation. *The Journal of the American Dental Association* 72 (1): 87–93.

11

Sealer-Based Obturations Using Bioceramics in Nonsurgical Root Canal Treatments

Garima Poddar[1,2], Ajay Bajaj[1,3], and Viresh Chopra[4,5,6]

[1] Diploma in Endodontics, Universität Jaume I (UJI), Castelló, Spain
[2] Dental Department, Shanti Memorial Hospital Pvt. Ltd., Cuttack, Odisha, India
[3] Private Practice, Mumbai, Maharashtra, India
[4] Endodontology, Oman Dental College, Muscat, Oman
[5] Adult Restorative Dentistry, Oman Dental College, Muscat, Oman
[6] Bart's London School of Medicine and Dentistry, Queen Mary University, London, UK

CONTENTS

Bioceramics in Endodontics, First Edition. Edited by Viresh Chopra.
© 2024 John Wiley & Sons, Inc. Published 2024 by John Wiley & Sons, Inc.
Companion website: www.wiley.com/go/chopra/bioceramicsinendodontics

11.1 Introduction

The objective of a root canal treatment is to avert invasion and proliferation of microbes by cleaning and obturating the root canal system of a tooth, tridimensionally, and also achieving a good seal both apically as well as coronally to prevent seepage of fluids and contaminants which could lead to a reinfection [1–3]. During an endodontic treatment, removing the infection-causing microorganisms, debris, and smear layer is important. Along with that, a proper obturation is equally critical, in order to prevent re-introduction of infection-causing factors into the canals. To realize the above-mentioned goals, obturation technique and the endodontic sealer used during the procedure plays an important role [2].

There has been a lot of progress in the field of endodontics, especially in the section of materials used in root canal treatments and retreatments, both surgically as well as nonsurgically. Bioceramics is one such material which has evolved a lot in the past few years [4].

Bioceramics can be classified into two broad categories:

1) Bioinert bioceramics like zirconia and alumina – these don't react with surroundings to which they are exposed.
2) Bioactive bioceramics – these react with the tissues in contact with the material. A material which is bioactive would be able to form a layer of hydroxyapatite

when in proximity to tissue fluids having contents like calcium and phosphates. Such bioceramic sealers would exhibit the following properties [5]:

a) Biocompatibility
b) Hermetic seal
c) Osteoinduction
d) Osteoconduction.

New bioceramic cements, which have become very popular in endodontics, can be used as a root canal sealer in routine root canal treatment cases as well as could be used in certain scenarios as a substitute of mineral trioxide aggregate (MTA) [6] Some of the multifold benefits of using the silicate sealers are [7–13]:

1) Noncytotoxic.
2) Bioceramic sealers expand while setting slightly (less than 0.2% of total volume expansion is encountered). The resorption of these sealers is not witnessed significantly.
3) Radiopaque.
4) pH of around 12.8 due to an alkaline environment it creates; the mineralization is good.
5) They are hydrophilic materials and lead to calcium phosphate formation on hydration, which provides strength.
6) A clinically favorable aspect of these sealers is that during unintentional over-obturation with bioceramics, the inflammatory response is very insignificant.

Due to the above properties, a sealer-based obturation is possible using bioceramic sealers where there is no requirement of increasing the proportion of gutta-percha as compared to the sealer [5].

In case of a sealer-based obturation, the role of a gutta-percha cone is to propel these silicate cements into gaps and ramifications of the root canal system, which have been cleaned properly during the shaping and cleaning phase. Also, since retreatment of a tooth filled using bioceramic cements is a laborious and difficult task, a core of gutta-percha proves to be helpful during removal of the obturating materials [5]. While performing root canal treatment of a tooth with splits or severe curvature of canals, many times the clinician finds warm vertical condesation (WVC) or continuous wave of condensation (CWC) techniques of obturation difficult to perform because of the inability of the tip of the down pack, backfill device, and even vertical pluggers to reach the desired depth inside the canals. In such cases, using a sealer-based obturation technique with a bioceramic sealer which could be injected into the canal is proving to be a good alternative in recent times. It further helps to learn that various randomized trials have documented the results that, a sealer-based obturation has been observed to be a good substitute to obturation using a resin-based sealer [14].

A single cone obturation technique has not been too successful in the recent past amongst clinicians due to the emergence of many voids that have been observed in canals filled with single cone with resin or zinc oxide eugenol-based sealers. But, with the advent of silicate cements as sealers, the technique has once again gained momentum [2, 15]. This chapter highlights the usage of the newer generation bioceramic sealer in three different cases of nonsurgical root canal treatments (NSRCTs) with the help of which root canal spaces could be obturated even in scenarios with conservative shaping; the splits could be filled with ease and also sealer propelled in other accessory canals/lateral canals. For a satisfactory obturation to take place, first and foremost, a thorough cleaning plays a crucial role. Removal of smear layer is also a key for achieving proper obturation of the root canal spaces. For this, use of irrigating solutions which could act on organic as well as inorganic parts of the debris is important during the endodontic treatment procedure. Since a single irrigating solution does not accomplish the task of removal of microbes, organic and inorganic debris, and smear layer, employing the use of more than one solution by developing a protocol for efficient and secure irrigation is needed [16].

The case reports elaborate the irrigation protocol followed during the root canal treatment of these teeth.

Performing the endodontic treatment procedure under rubber dam isolation further helps in being able to provide a contamination-free field of work.

11.2 Case 1

11.2.1 Patient Information

- Age: 69
- Gender: Male
- Medical history: Type 2 diabetic, on medication for the same. Diabetes in control after medication.

11.2.2 Details of the Tooth

Identification: Tooth number 35 (mandibular left second premolar)

Dental history: Patient reported with pain and tenderness in mandibular left posterior region for 15 days.

Clinical Examination Findings: On clinical examination, it was observed that the area of concern had a long span fixed prosthesis. Teeth numbers 34 and 35 were tender on percussion. The pain was sharp in nature. The fixed prosthesis was ill-fitting and had a crack. Patient had a traumatic occlusion due to faulty prosthesis.

11.2.3 Radiographic Evaluation of Tooth Number 35 Revealed the Following

Radiographic evaluation revealed the following:

1) Periodontal ligament widening was present.
2) The tooth was a taurodont tooth with one canal splitting into two in the middle third region of the root, that is, having a 1–2 configuration/type IV Weine's configuration.
3) Slight periapical radiolucency was also observed on the radiograph in relation to the tooth.
4) Tooth number 34 has a horizontal root fracture (Figure 11.1).

11.2.4 Diagnosis

Pulpal – Symptomatic irreversible pulpitis
   Periapical – Symptomatic apical periodontitis

11.3 Treatment Plan

1) Extraction of fractured tooth number 34.
2) NSRCT of tooth number 35.
3) Fixed partial denture (FPD) to be redone by referring dentist.
4) Dental implant planned for 34 regions after healing and bone deposition has satisfactorily taken place.
5) Recall: Follow-up recalls planned at six months and one year after the treatment is completed.

Figure 11.1 Preoperative radiograph.

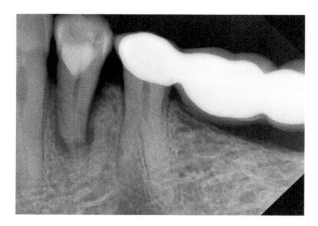

11.4 Treatment Done

The FPD was removed and tooth was isolated using rubber dam isolation. Access preparation was done and splits were negotiated using 8K and 10K hand files. Proper tactile examination and detailed study of the preoperative radiograph proved to be helpful.

11.4.1 Instrumentation Protocol

Coronal flaring was done using One Flare file (Micro-Mega, France). The working length was then determined with the help of an electronic apex locator and it was also confirmed with a radiograph. The canals were instrumented with a 10K file until it became loose in both the splits. The file was precurved in the apical third, so that it easily follows the natural canal curvature. Gentle, watch-winding motion was the technique used for shaping with hand files. After withdrawal of file each time from the canal, irrigation was done using sodium hypochlorite. Recapitulation was done with one size smaller file to maintain patency of the canal to the working length. Glide path preparation was done with the help of gyromatic hand piece – K400 (Dontics, Bombay Dental and Surgical) and 15 number K file. Once the glide path was prepared, it ensured smooth gliding of the file to the desired working length. Irrigation was given importance throughout shaping, and was performed after each step of instrumentation. Shaping of both the canals/splits was done with Hero gold files (Micro-Mega, France). The main trunk was shaped to 25-06% and rest of the canal till working length was shaped to 25-04%. Conservative shaping was done in order to preserve dentin where possible.

11.4.2 Irrigation Protocol

Throughout shaping, 5.25% sodium hypochlorite was used after each file. Side vented 30-gauge needles were used for irrigation.

After shaping, the following protocol in each canal was used for irrigation and activation of irrigants:

1) 17% ethylene diamine tetra acetic acid (EDTA) – 1 ml per canal – ultrasonic activation with EndoUltra (Vista).
2) Distilled water used to flush the canals.
3) 5.25% sodium hypochlorite – intracanal heating of sodium hypochlorite – ultrasonic activation (four such cycles repeated per canal).
4) Distilled water.

11.4.3 Obturation Protocol

Cone fit intraoral radiograph was made and master cones were selected (Figure 11.2).

Canals were dried with paper points. Care was taken not to dehydrate the canals, since the sealer to be used was chosen to be bioceramic.

One split was blocked by inserting a paper point and gutta-percha cone was inserted in the other split, and then the paper point in the other split was also replaced with cone. A sealer-based obturation was done using bioceramic sealer-CeraSeal (Meta Biomed). The technique used was as follows:

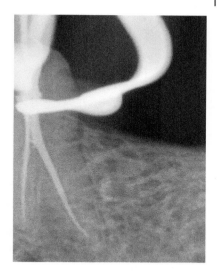

Figure 11.2 Cone fit radiograph.

1) One split was blocked by inserting a paper point.
2) CeraSeal was injected in the other split.
3) Gutta-percha cone was inserted in the other split.
4) Paper point from the other split was removed and CeraSeal was injected in this split.
5) Then gutta-percha cone was inserted in this split.
6) The obturation was vertically compacted by employing a continuous wave of compaction technique using EQ-V (Meta Biomed), as this sealer is heat compatible. Care was taken to limit the extent of inserting the down pack tip to the beginning of the middle third

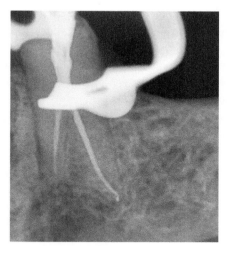

Figure 11.3 Immediate post-op radiograph.

of the canal length. On the immediate postoperative radiograph (Figure 11.3), it can be seen that there was some sealer flow due to the vertical compaction of the obturating material, which helped in attaining better seal in the apical third.

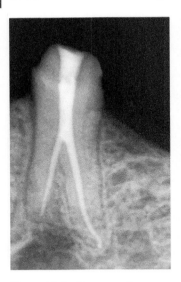

Figure 11.4 Postoperative radiograph.

11.4.4 Post Endodontic Restoration

Composite was used for post endodontic restoration using layering technique (Figure 11.4)

The patient was referred to referring dentist who fabricated and placed a fixed partial denture in that region.

11.4.5 Rationale on the Treatment Protocol and the Material Used

Tooth number 35 was part of an FPD, so crown preparation had been done previously for that tooth. While preforming the endodontic treatment, care was taken to be as conservative as practical in order to retain the healthy dentin as tooth structure as possible. It was also taken into consideration that after the endodontic treatment, once again a fixed prosthesis was planned for this tooth.

The shaping was also done conservatively, with final apical diameter of 25-04% for both the splits.

Due to the acceptable properties mentioned before, conservative preparations and easy obturation of the canal configuration, sealer-based obturation using a bioceramic sealer was chosen as the technique for tooth number 35.

11.5 Learning Objectives for the Readers

1) Negotiation of the canals and instrumentation of such canal configuration is challenging at times. Therefore, a proper instrumentation plan should be laid down in order to execute the instrumentation successfully.
2) Obturating such a canal configuration is even more difficult as the obturating materials are soft, while the shaping files are made up of metal and hence are stiff. The obturating technique mentioned in the case report makes the obturation of splits easier.

11.6 Case 2

11.6.1 Patient Information

- Age: 40
- Gender: Female
- Medical history: Not relevant

11.6.2 Details of the Tooth

- Identification: Mandibular second molar of left side – tooth number 37
- Dental history: Patient had history of extraction of tooth number 36 four years back.
  Patient also complained of deviation of the path of closure of TMJ.
  She also gave history of bruxism when she felt stress.
- History of restoration in tooth number 37.

11.6.2.1 Clinical Examination Findings

The patient had faulty occlusion in the left quadrant, with tooth number 36 missing and tooth number 37 titled in the missing tooth space (Figure 11.5). The tooth was tender to percussion. She had a deviated path of closure of TMJ and also had a tendency of shifting her occlusion frequently.

She complained of severe and continuous pain in the mandibular left posterior region for one month which was radiating to the temple on the left side and the ear as well. The patient was unable to localize the source of pain as it was radiating and sharp in nature. Cold test using endo ice– Endo-Frost (Roeko, Coltene)– was performed for tooth number 37 (Figure 11.6). On application of the cold stimulus, there was spontaneous sharp pain response which lingered for more than five seconds.

11.6.2.2 Preoperative Radiological Assessment

The preoperative CBCT report (Figures 11.5, 11.7, 11.8 and 11.9) revealed the following:

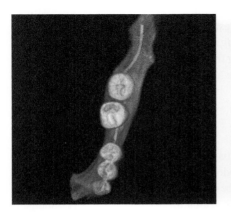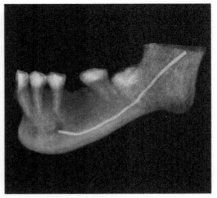

Figure 11.5 Three dimensional preoperative cone beam computed tomography (CBCT) images of tooth number 37.

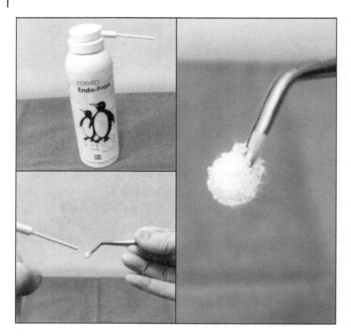

Figure 11.6 Cold sensitivity test using endo-ice.

1) Tooth number 37 was mesially inclined (Figure 11.5).
2) No significant crown or root fracture was noted.
3) Presence of sclerotic area medial to mesial root of 37. Area measured approximately 14.7 mm (SI) and extended inferiorly from the crestal to superior border of the infra alveolar nerve (IAN). Anteriorly, the area measured approximately 6.6 mm.
4) Tooth number 37 had a radiopaque restoration involving enamel and dentin.
5) Tooth number 38 was impacted having a deep-seated impaction and the mesial cusp of tooth number 38 lay abutting the cervical third of the distal root of 37.
6) IAN lay in very close proximity to the apical third of the roots of 38 on the lingual aspect.

11.6.3 Diagnosis

Pulpal – Symptomatic irreversible pulpitis
  Periapical – Symptomatic apical periodontitis
  The sclerotic area medial to 37 could not be diagnosed with affirmation (Figure 11.10).
  Differential diagnosis for sclerotic area (i) Idiopathic osteosclerosis. (ii) Condensing osteitis [17, 18]

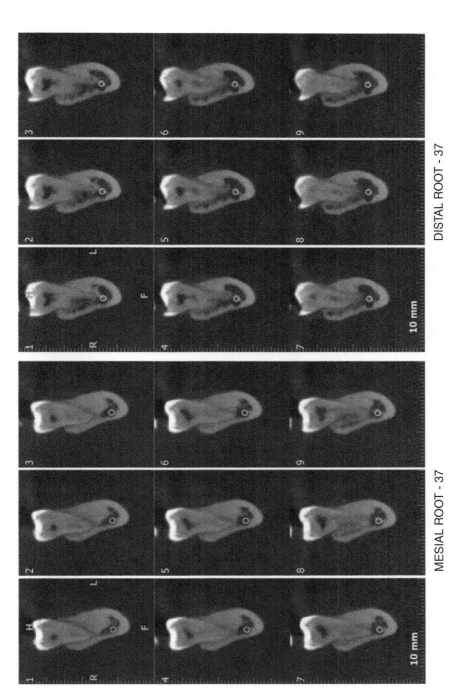

MESIAL ROOT - 37

DISTAL ROOT - 37

10 mm

10 mm

Figure 11.7   CBCT images of mesial and distal roots of tooth number 37.

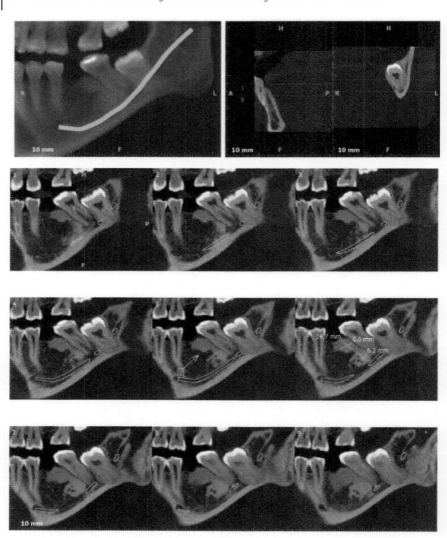

1 : SCLEROTIC MASS MEDIAL TO 37 REGION

Figure 11.8 CBCT images showing sclerotic area mesial to 37.

11.7 Treatment Plan

NSRCT of tooth number 37.

Follow-ups at frequent intervals to observe situation of 38 as patient was unwilling for a surgical treatment unless pain does not subside.

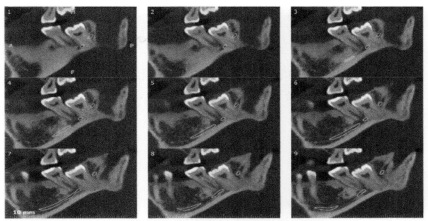

IMPACTED 38 AND ITS RELATION TO 37

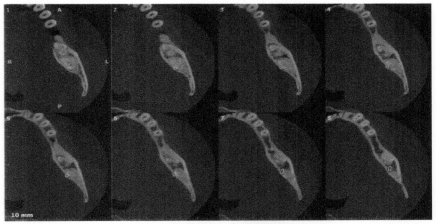

AXIAL SECTIONS - LEFT MANDIBLE

Figure 11.9 Axial section CBCT for tooth number 37.

Periodic follow-ups for the sclerotic area medial to tooth number 37 to observe if the sclerosis is showing growth or if its regressing.

Recall:
- First recall at two weeks of treatment.
- Second recall after one month.
- Third recall at six months interval.

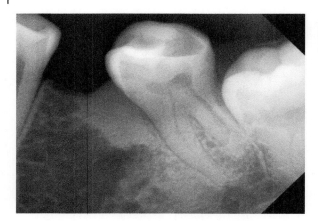

Figure 11.10 Intraoral-periapical radiograph of tooth number 37, showing the sclerotic mass mesial to 37.

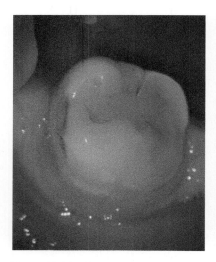

Figure 11.11 Preoperative clinical image of tooth 37.

11.8 Treatment Done

Local anesthesia was administered (2% lignocaine with 1 : 80000 adrenaline) using an anesthesia delivery device – Star Pen (Woodpecker, China) for controlled delivery of anesthetic solution. Tooth number 37 was isolated using rubber dam and old composite restoration was removed. Access preparation was completed and three canals were located. The tooth was observed to have a C- shaped canal configuration. According to Fan et al., it was C2 configuration [19–21].

11.8.1 Instrumentation Protocol

Pre-instrumentation irrigation was followed by preflaring of the canals using One Flare file (Coltene-Micro-Mega, France).

Negotiation of mesial canals was done with 8 number K file whereas a 10 number K file was used to negotiate the distal canal (Figure 11.12). Working length determination was done using electronic apex locator of endo motor integrated with apex locator (EndoMatic, Woodpecker, China). Manual instrumentation was

Figure 11.12 Working length radiograph.

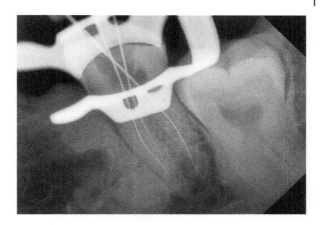

done with 10 number K file until it was loose in all the three canals to desired working length. While performing manual instrumentation, precurving K files and giving it a gradual curvature in the apical third proved to be helpful in this case. Slight teasing motion along with watch-winding technique was utilized for this step. Glide path preparation was done with One G files (Micro-Mega, France). Crown down technique was carried out, and middle third was shaped first to 6% taper followed by which apical third was prepared to 4% taper. Instrumentation was performed using Hero gold files (Micro-Mega, France) to size 30–06% until middle third and 25-4% in the apical third using crown down technique of shaping. Irrigation at each step during shaping is of great importance in order to prevent debris getting collected in the canals. Recapitulation was done using 10 number K file after each rotary file usage also for maintenance of patency of the canal throughout the working length.

11.8.2 Irrigation Protocol

5.25% sodium hypochlorite was used in the canals during shaping procedure.

Once instrumentation was completed, distilled water was used to flush the canals.

1 ml of 17% EDTA liquid was injected in the canals which was then activated using ultrasonic tips (Woodpecker, China) for 50–60 seconds in each canal. Distilled water was used to flush out the EDTA liquid from the canals. 5.25% sodium hypochlorite was introduced in the canals, and the solution was then ultrasonically activated. Flexible Irriflex needles (Produits Dentaires, Switzerland) were used to deliver the irrigation material inside the root canal. Fresh batch of sodium hypochlorite was introduced in each canal three times, following which ultrasonic activation was done. Distilled water was used for final rinse.

11.8.3 Obturation Protocol

Master cones were selected for all the shaped canals (Figure 11.13). Paper points were then used to dry the canals. Overdrying was avoided as bioceramic cement was the sealer of choice for this case. CeraSeal (Meta Biomed, Korea), which is a bioceramic sealer was injected in all the canals, following which master cones were inserted. The extent of sealer flow and gutta-percha in the canals was confirmed with a radiograph (Figure 11.14).

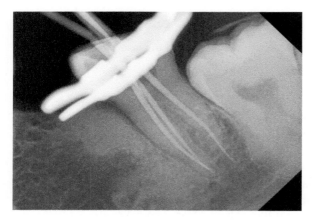

Figure 11.13 Cone fit radiograph of tooth 37.

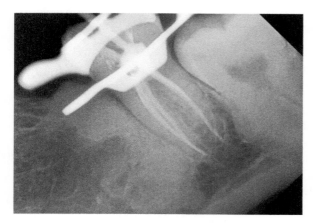

Figure 11.14 Immediate postop radiograph.

Figure 11.15 Postobturation clinical image of access cavity of tooth number 37 showing C2 configuration.

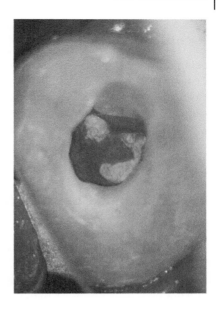

Figure 11.16 Postop radiograph after core buildup with composites.

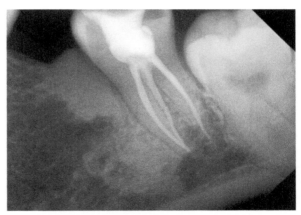

Vertical compaction technique was performed using the down pack tip of EQ-V (Meta Biomed, Korea). The C2 canal configuration could be appreciated (Figure 11.15). Core buildup was done using warm composites (Figure 11.16).

11.8.4 Post Endodontic Phase

Correction of traumatic occlusion has been planned in future. A night guard has been delivered to the patient for relief from her bruxism habit.

11.8.5 Rationale on the Treatment Protocol and the Material Used

Being an injectable sealer with good flow, choosing a bioceramic sealer for a C-shaped anatomy is a justifiable choice. Since patient had suffered severe pain, bioceramic sealers exhibit properties of biocompatibility and, clinically, the patient does not experience pain in most of the cases, a sealer-based obturation was chosen as the technique for this case. In addition, other properties like expansion of hydraulic cements on setting works in the favour of using these materials as sealers during obturations.

11.9 Learning Objectives for the Readers

1) Diagnosis of a case properly and then planning the treatment is of utmost importance in order to perform a satisfactory treatment.
2) For optimum usage of the materials and techniques, it's vital to have a sound knowledge of the science behind them.
3) Thorough irrigation is of high value in order to clean and disinfect the root canal system and then seal them well.
4) Traumatic occlusion could culminate in endodontically compromised teeth and, at the same time, also decrease the quality of living of the patient.

11.10 Case 3

11.10.1 Patient Information

- Age: 27
- Gender: Female
- Medical history: Non-relevant

11.10.2 Details of the Tooth

- Identification: Maxillary first premolar of left side – tooth number 24
- Dental history: Patient complained of occasional pain in the tooth. The pain was dull aching in nature. She also complained of food impaction in that region.
- Clinical examination findings:
  - Cold test – there was pain which lasted for more than five seconds on application of a cold stimulus using endo ice (Roeko, Coltene).
  - Deep disto-proximal carious lesion was present involving the pulp.
  - Mild tenderness on percussion was present.

11.10.3 Preoperative Radiological Assessment

Preoperative radiograph (Figure 11.17) revealed the following details:

Deep proximal caries extending to enamel, dentin, and pulp of tooth number 24 was seen on the intraoral periapical radiograph.

1) Periodontal widening was observed in the apical area.
2) Very thin canals were observed on the radiograph.

11.10.4 Diagnosis

Pulpal – Symptomatic irreversible pulpitis.
Periapical – Symptomatic apical periodontitis.

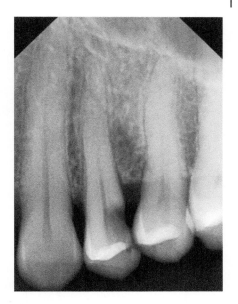

Figure 11.17 Preoperative intraoral radiograph of tooth number 24.

11.11 Treatment plan

- Root canal treatment of tooth number 24 followed by post and core and full coverage, zirconia crown.
- Recall: Next recall after six months.

11.12 Treatment Done

Local anesthesia was administered – local infiltration with 2% lignocaine with 1 : 80,000 concentration adrenaline. Rubber dam isolation was done. As a part of pre-endodontic restoration, the disto-proximal wall was built using liquid dam (Figure 11.18). Two canals were found, namely buccal and palatal.

11.12.1 Instrumentation Protocol

Since the canals were very thin to begin with, coronal flaring was done using One Flare file (Coltene, Micro-Mega, France). Since the size of this file is 25-09%, it prevents excessive removal of pericervical dentin.

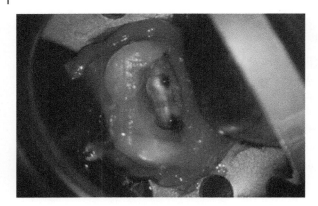

Figure 11.18 Intraoral clinical image of tooth number 24 showing rubber dam isolation and access cavity preparation.

Smaller K files used to negotiate and shape the canals were 6K, 8K, and 10K. The instrumentation technique with hand files used was passive step back technique and balanced force technique. The hand files were given gentle precurvature in the apical third to facilitate its smooth progression in the canal, following the natural canal curvature. Glide path preparation was done using One G file (Coltene-Micro-Mega, France). After withdrawal of each K file or rotary instrument, thorough irrigation with sodium hypochlorite was performed. Recapitulation to maintain patency of the canal throughout the working length was done. Shaping was done with 2Shape files (Coltene-Micro-Mega, France) until 25 number size and 4% taper using crown down technique.

11.12.2 Irrigation Protocol

Irrigation was done using side vented polymer needles- IrriFlex (Produits Dentaires, Switzerland), 5.25% sodium hypochlorite was used to irrigate the canals throughout the procedure of shaping. Once shaping was achieved, dedicated time was given to irrigation and activation of irrigating solutions in the following order:

1) Distilled water to flush out the canals.
2) 17% EDTA liquid was injected in both buccal and mesial canals and the solution was activated using ultrasonic tips (Woodpecker, China). This was carried out for approximately one minute per canal.
3) Distilled water was utilized to flush the canals.
4) 5.25% sodium hypochlorite (Cerkamed, Poland) was injected in the canals and solution was ultrasonically activated. This step was repeated three times per canal.

11.12.3 Obturation Protocol

Master cone was selected and checked for true tug-back (Figure 11.20).

Paper points were used in both the canals to get rid of the excess moisture (Figure 11.19), but importance was given not to overdry the canals, as bioceramic sealers exhibit better setting and optimum properties when the canals are not overdry.

Single cone with bioceramic cement as sealer was chosen as the technique for this case. Bioceramic sealer, CeraSeal (Meta Biomed) was injected in the canals. During this step care should be taken to prevent extrusion of the material periapically since these sealers have a good flow. Care needs to be taken that the tip of the syringe does not get wedged inside the canal. The applicator tip of the syringe was

Figure 11.19 Clinical image showing drying of canals using paper points.

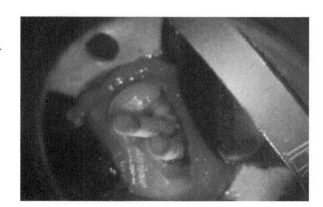

Figure 11.20 Cone fit radiograph

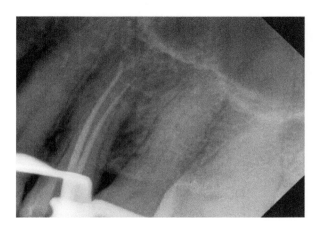

kept 2 mm short of the working length. The syringe was withdrawn simultaneously as the material was being injected in the canals in order to prevent extrusion of the sealer beyond the apex. Then, the selected master cones were inserted into the canals. The position of master cones was confirmed with the help of radiographs also (Figure 11.20). The cones were seared off with a heated device at the canal orifice level, and a slight compaction with a vertical plugger was done. Interesting root canal anatomy got filled up. Two lateral canals could be appreciated on the immediate postop radiographs (Figures 11.21 and 11.22).

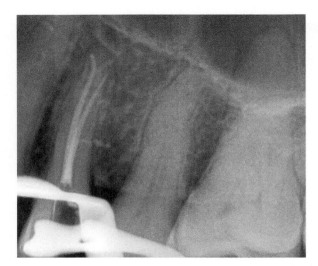

Figure 11.21 Immediate postop straight view.

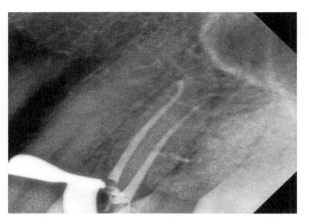

Figure 11.22 Immediate postop angulated view.

11.12.4 Post Endo Restorative Phase

Post space was prepared immediately after obturation, as once the bioceramic sealer sets it would have become a difficult task to remove it for post space preparation. Patient was recalled after two days. At this point, fiber postTenax, size 1.1 (Coltene) was placed and core buildup was done using warm composites. A full coverage zirconia crown was fabricated and cemented to tooth number 24.

11.12.5 Rationale on the Treatment Protocol and the Material Used

To begin with, the canals were very thin and 6K number file had to be used to negotiate the canals. Thus, in this case, the final shaping of the apical third was done with 25-04% file. For such cases, where the shaping is conservative, using thin gauge polymer, double side vented needles served to be efficient as the irrigating solution is able to reach a greater depth in the canals with ease.

Also, using a sealer-based obturation with single cone and bioceramic sealer proved to be convenient. Since cleaning of the canals was satisfactory, accessory canals also got filled up with hydraulic sealer.

11.13 Learning Objectives for the Readers

1) Performing thorough irrigation using appropriate and efficient irrigating solutions is an important aspect of root canal treatment. In addition, when using a sealer-based obturation, a proper flow of sealer to every nook and corner of the root canal space is highly dependent on cleaning of the root canal system.
2) While obturating a root canal with bioceramics, overdrying should not be done as it is a hydrophilic material whose setting is better when canals are not too dry.
3) Side vented needles made of polymer are more flexible and their double side vents are at the same level, which provides better flow of solutions inside the root canal system.

11.14 Discussion

There has been a rise in the employment of sealer-based obturation technique using bioceramic sealers by clinicians in recent times. Silicate cements have shown good results clinically for different endodontic treatment procedures. Clinically, the bioceramic cements have shown higher level performances compared to other materials which we have used for many decades. [22].

Before commencing with a root canal treatment, a thorough knowledge, examination, and radiograph-based diagnosis is important to yield good results of the treatment in future. A detailed treatment planning taking into consideration the prosthetic phase of the tooth concerned is very crucial. For that, having a multidisciplinary approach and discussing the details of a particular case with the prosthodontic team is very important.

When carrying out a NSRCT, shaping, cleaning, and efficient obturation, all play a major role in good prognosis of that endodontically treated tooth.

A sealer-based obturation with the help of bioceramic sealers helps in creating very few voids inside the root canal space. So, achieving a good hermetic seal in the apical third of the tooth becomes easier. Furthermore, since the bioceramic sealer expands slightly on or after setting, it further prevents chances of percolation of fluids or contamination into the tooth [7–11].

References

1 Pontoriero, D., Madaro, G., Vanagolli, V. et al. (2021). Sealing ability of a bioceramic sealer used in combination with cold and warm obturation techniques. *Journal of Osseointegration.* 13 (4): 248–255.

2 Mannocci, F., Innocenti, M., Bertelli, E., and Ferrari, M. (1999). Dye leakage and SEM study of roots obturated with Thermafill and dentin bonding agent. *Dental Traumatology.* 15 (2): 60–64.

3 Ingle, J. and Bakland, L. (2002). *Endodontics*, 5e. Hamilton: BC Decker.

4 Raghavendra, S.S., Jadhav, G.R., Gathani, K.M., and Kotadia, P. (2017). Bioceramics in endodontics–a review. *Journal of Istanbul University Faculty of Dentistry.* 51 (3 Suppl 1): S128.

5 Kohli, M.R. and Karabucak, B. (2019). Bioceramic usage in endodontics. *American Association of Endoodntics* July.

6 Krell, K.F. and Wefel, J.S. (1984). A calcium phosphate cement root canal sealer—scanning electron microscopic analysis. *Journal of Endodontics.* 10 (12): 571–576.

7 Viapiana, R., Flumignan, D., Guerreiro-Tanomaru, J. et al. (2014). Physicochemical and mechanical properties of zirconium oxide and niobium oxide modified P ortland cement-based experimental endodontic sealers. *International Endodontic Journal.* 47 (5): 437–448.

8 Erdemir, A., Adanir, N., and Belli, S. (2003). In vitro evaluation of the dissolving effect of solvents on root canal sealers. *Journal of Oral Science.* 45 (3): 123–126.

9 Gandolfi, M. and Prati, C. (2010). MTA and F-doped MTA cements used as sealers with warm gutta-percha. Long-term study of sealing ability. *International Endodontic Journal.* 43 (10): 889–901.

10 Morgental, R.D., Vier-Pelisser, F.V., Oliveira, S.D. et al. (2011). Antibacterial activity of two MTA-based root canal sealers. *International Endodontic Journal.* 44 (12): 1128–1133.

11 Tanomaru-Filho, M., Silveira, G.F., Tanomaru, J.M.G., and Bier, C.A.S. (2007). Evaluation of the thermoplasticity of different gutta-percha cones and Resilon®. *Australian Endodontic Journal.* 33 (1): 23–26.

12 Costa, B.C., Guerreiro-Tanomaru, J.M., Bosso-Martelo, R. et al. (2018). Ytterbium oxide as radiopacifier of calcium silicate-based cements. Physicochemical and biological properties. *Brazilian Dental Journal.* 29: 452–458.

13 Prüllage, R.-K., Urban, K., Schäfer, E., and Dammaschke, T. (2016). Material properties of a tricalcium silicate–containing, a mineral trioxide aggregate–containing, and an epoxy resin–based root canal sealer. *Journal of Endodontics.* 42 (12): 1784–1788.

14 Kim, J.-h., Cho, S.-Y., Choi, Y. et al. (2022). Clinical efficacy of sealer-based obturation using calcium silicate sealers: a randomized clinical trial. *Journal of Endodontics.* 48 (2): 144–151.

15 Celikten, B., Uzuntas, C.F., Orhan, A.I. et al. (2015). Micro-CT assessment of the sealing ability of three root canal filling techniques. *Journal of Oral Science.* 57 (4): 361–366.

16 Topbas, C. and Adiguzel, O. (2017). Endodontic irrigation solutions: a review: endodontic irrigation solutions. *International Dental Research.* 7 (3): 54–61.

17 Sisman, Y., Ertas, E.T., Ertas, H., and Sekerci, A.E. (2011). The frequency and distribution of idiopathic osteosclerosis of the jaw. *European Journal of Dentistry.* 5 (04): 409–414.

18 Al-Habib, M.A. (2022). Prevalence and pattern of idiopathic osteosclerosis and condensing osteitis in a Saudi subpopulation. *Cureus.* 14 (2).

19 Fernandes, M., De Ataide, I., and Wagle, R. (2014). C-shaped root canal configuration: a review of literature. *Journal of Conservative Dentistry: JCD.* 17 (4): 312.

20 Fan, B., Cheung, G.S., Fan, M. et al. (2004). C-shaped canal system in mandibular second molars: part I—anatomical features. *Journal of Endodontics.* 30 (12): 899–903.

21 Fan, W., Fan, B., Gutmann, J.L., and Fan, M. (2008). Identification of a C-shaped canal system in mandibular second molars—part III: anatomic features revealed by digital subtraction radiography. *Journal of Endodontics.* 34 (10): 1187–1190.

22 Camilleri, J., Atmeh, A., Li, X., and Meschi, N. (2022). Present status and future directions: Hydraulic materials for endodontic use. *International Endodontic Journal.* 55: 710–777.

12

BioConeless Obturation

Francesca Cerutti[1] and Calogero Bugea[2]

[1] *Private Practice, Lovere, Italy*
[2] *Private Practice, Gallipoli, Italy*

CONTENTS

12.1 Introduction

The aim of 3D obturation is to create a compact, homogeneous, and three-dimensional defense against the eventual invasion of microorganisms into a root canal system that has been properly shaped and cleaned [1]. Consequently, canal obturation is currently considered a crucial step to make a root canal treatment (RCT) successful in the long term. Several root canal obturation techniques based on gutta-percha and sealers have been proposed over the years [2, 3]. These techniques can be divided in two categories: cold techniques and warm techniques. Cold techniques, such as the single cone technique and

Bioceramics in Endodontics, First Edition. Edited by Viresh Chopra.
© 2024 John Wiley & Sons, Inc. Published 2024 by John Wiley & Sons, Inc.
Companion website: www.wiley.com/go/chopra/bioceramicsinendodontics

the lateral condensation, have shown poor sealing capacity in vitro, mainly because of the insufficient adaptation capacity of the cold gutta-percha to the canal space [4]. Moreover, the voids created cannot be fully compensated by the big amount of sealer needed in these techniques compared to warm ones [5]. On the contrary, warm techniques, which exploit the thermal properties of the gutta-percha, allow for a better adaptation to the root canal anatomy and thus ensure a stronger sealing ability [6, 7].

Thermoplasticized gutta-percha has been found to be able to flow into irregular spaces, such as isthmuses and lateral canals and, consequently, is considered a more effective method to fill the root canal space [8].

The gutta-percha can be brought into the root canal as a point that is subsequently heated by means of dedicated heat carriers, then the softened material is packed by means of pluggers. The remaining part of the root canal is then back filled with thermoplasticized gutta-percha extruded by means of devices like Obtura III Max (Obtura Spartan, Algonquin, IL) or Fast Fill (Eighteeth, Changzhou City, China).

An alternative way to do a warm obturation is by extruding directly the thermoplasticized gutta-percha into the root canal previously dressed with sealer. When the thermoplasticized gutta-percha is extruded into a root canal dressed with a bioceramic sealer, it is called BioConeless.

Root canal obturation by injection of thermoplasticized gutta-percha was first described by Yee et al. in 1977 [9]. This technique is based on a direct injection of thermoplasticized gutta-percha inside the canal by means of a dedicated gutta-percha injector to reach a complete endodontic space filling [9, 10]. Several studies have underlined the efficacy of this technique in filling the endodontic space [11, 12]. Encouraging results have emerged from in vitro studies investigating the efficacy of canal obturation by injection-molded thermoplasticized gutta-percha (ITG) [11–13]. On the other hand, to date, few clinical studies are available in literature on the outcomes of teeth filled with this technique; the existing papers reported complete healing rates ranging from 93.1% to 100% after observation periods ranging between six months and three years [10, 14, 15].

According to the literature, the injection of thermoplasticized gutta-percha has several advantages if compared to the other warm techniques; in fact, the procedure is time-saving, it allows obtaining a good filling of the root canal system, and it is also able to fill complex anatomies (Figure 12.1a–d). The reported disadvantages are the risk of incomplete filling or overfilling [10, 13–17].

The injection of thermoplasticized gutta-percha has been associated to zinc oxide eugenol (ZOE) sealers for a long time (since ZOE sealers were broadly used for warm vertical compaction techniques due to their wide availability, low cost, and good chemical and physical properties), but it can be used also with resin-based sealers [18, 19].

(a)   (b)

(c)   (d)

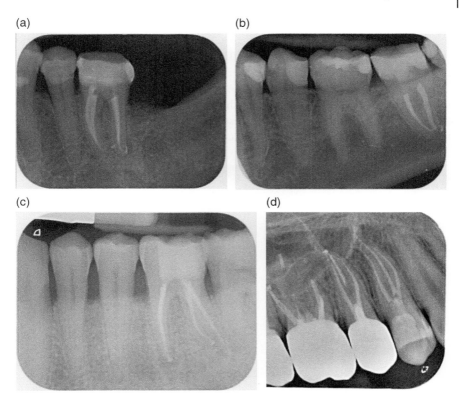

Figure 12.1 (a–d) Particular anatomies that can be treated with the bioconeless technique.

12.2 Why BioConeless?

The spread of calcium silicate–based sealers, whose biocompatibility and excellent properties were reported by several articles, are described by some authors as the future of root canal sealers, even if at the moment there is no evidence of their superiority in terms of success rate with respect to other sealers [20–23]. Calcium silicate–based sealers were first formulated in order to be used with cold techniques, the single cone technique in particular, or lateral compaction technique [24].

In root canals with constant taper and where the fitting of the gutta-percha point is precise, the single cone technique with bioceramic sealer works very well, because the point acts as a piston that pushes the sealer laterally, with a declinate but efficient wedge effect [25–27]. Conversely, sometimes, root canals have an oval shape (i.e. the distal roots of lower molars in the presence of a root canal whose shape is like a double-barreled shotgun) or we are not able to reach the apex due to the presence of iatrogenic blocks, apical deltas, broken instruments, or abrupt apical curvatures: in these cases, the hydraulic push generated by the gutta-percha point on the sealer is not efficient and the root canal filling ends up being insufficient [28–31].

In the case shown in Figures 12.2–12.6, a single cone technique with calcium silicate–based sealer was used to seal the distal root of this lower molar. The clinician was not satisfied with the result obtained with the bioactive sealer because the anatomy of the root was not correctly filled. At this point, the vertical

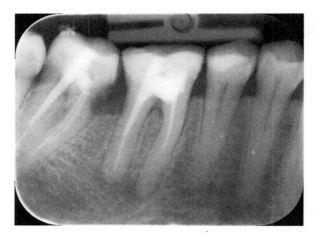

Figure 12.2 A patient came to our attention complaining about pain on chewing on tooth 4.6. She was diagnosed with symptomatic apical periodontitis and the treatment plan was to do a nonsurgical retreatment on the tooth.

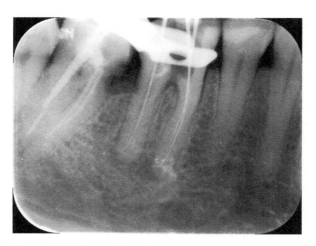

Figure 12.3 The existing filling material was removed and the glide path was done, as confirmed by the intraoperative X-ray.

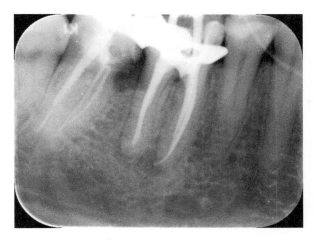

Figure 12.4 The tooth was filled with the single cone and calcium silicate–based sealer, but the X-ray showed an insufficient filing of the distal canal.

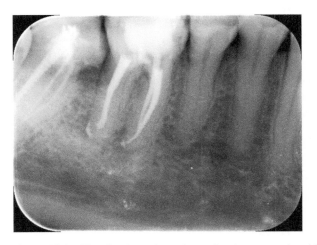

Figure 12.5 The distal canal was immediately retreated and filled with the vertical warm compaction technique.

warm compaction of the gutta-percha was necessary in order to achieve correct filling of the root canal system. This clinical case confirms that there is not a single technique that can be used successfully to fill the root canal system in every case, but that we need to know several techniques in order to manage correctly all the clinical scenarios that we face [32].

Not every bioactive sealer can be used with warm techniques: in fact, the presence of heat tends to limit the flow of the material and to increase the setting reaction due to the evaporation of water [16].

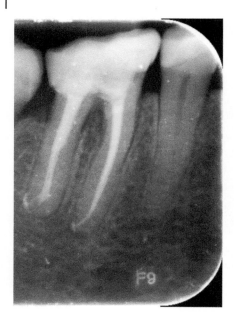

Figure 12.6 2 years follow-up.

The increasing request for a material to be used with warm gutta-percha compaction techniques led some manufacturers to modify the composition of their sealers, making them heat-compatible; premixed sealers containing propylene glycol instead of water, characterized by a high flow ability, were developed for this aim.

If we used a water-based calcium silicate–based sealer, the temperature of the tip of the back-fill device (ranging between 60 and 80 °C, according to the brand of the device chosen) would crystallize the sealer in contact with the tip, causing a total or partial block of the extrusion of gutta-percha [33]. On the other hand, when using propylene glycol calcium silicate–based sealers, the heat is not able to cause the immediate crystallization of the product, making it possible to use heat inside of the root canal.

According to Drukteinis and Camilleri, "the unique properties of the highly flowable and dimensionally stable hydraulic calcium silicate–based sealers, the down-pack procedure became easier and should not be performed so precisely in comparison to cases when conventional sealers are used." Since "the hydraulic calcium silicate–based sealers are dimensionally stable and flow into all root canal irregularities, isthmuses, and dentinal tubules, therefore, the thickness of the sealer layer is not important to ensure the high-quality obturation, even if the minimal condensation to softened gutta-percha is applied" [24]. In addition, a microleakage study by De Angelis et al. reported promising results of the warm continuous wave of condensation combined with a bioceramic sealer [13, 34].

Other ex vivo studies by Abdellatif et al. [16] and Pontoriero et al. [17] reported good performances of bioceramic sealers combined with warm techniques thanks to the capability of the sealer to fill lateral canals and to obtain good scores in microleakage studies.

12.2.1 BioConeless: Indications

There are few indications reported for using the BioConeless technique. It is not necessary to have a specific taper to fill the root canals with the BioConeless technique, since it can be done with every kind of preparation. However, the apical size that is considered as a cut-off is 0.7 mm. In foramina larger than that, it is not advised to use the BioConeless technique, because the risk of extrusion of gutta-percha and sealer into the periodontium would be extremely high [35].

In the initial treatments, the BioConeless technique is particularly indicated when it is not possible to find a gutta-percha point that is adequately fitting into the root canal, or the gutta percha point has not a good tug back or remains excessively short to the working length.

Some typical situation in which the BioConeless technique is extremely useful is that of apical deltas or abrupt apical curvatures [18, 34]: when this happens, a high pressure is required to push the gutta-percha and sealers into the areas that have been cleaned by the irrigants, and the insertion of warm gutta-percha into the root canals makes the filling phase easier and more predictable (Figure 12.7).

Figure 12.7 Apical deltas and canal confluences can be easily filled with the BioConeless technique.

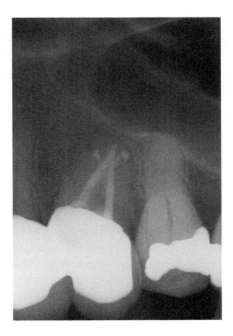

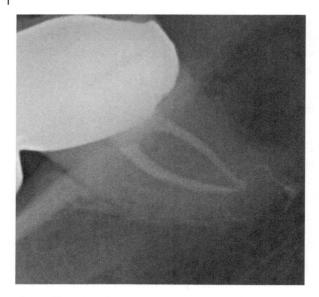

Figure 12.8 The force applied on the root canal walls by the warm gutta-percha can push the sealer apically.

Another clinical situation in which the BioConeless technique is extremely effective and time saving is that of confluences: once the main root canal has been filled (with any technique), the secondary canal can be easily and quickly filled with bioceramic sealer and BioConeless technique [34]; in some of these cases, the pressure of the gutta-percha on the confluent canal will further push the bioceramic sealer to the apical area filling even more the confluence (Figure 12.8).

In case of lower molars with double-barreled shotgun-shaped canals, the pressure applied by a single cone on the bioceramic sealer is insufficient to fill the entire anatomy; for this reason, the BioConeless technique can be used [34]. If one still wants to use the single cone technique, it is possible to use a single cone and then fill with the back-fill device the space left between the master cone and the root canal walls, ensuring an adequate push to the bioceramic sealer to flow into the root canal system.

In retreatments, the BioConeless technique can help when we find a separated instrument that we cannot bypass or we bypassed with a lot of effort: even in this case, the pressure applied on the sealer by the warm gutta-percha will be greater than the one applied with a single cone (Figures 12.9–12.11).

The presence of a stripping in a root is a major indication for the BioConeless technique because it will permit to seal with gutta-percha and sealer the area of

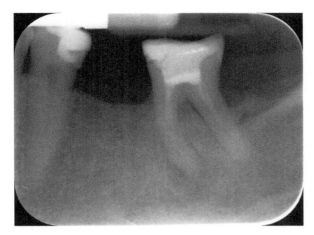

Figure 12.9 A patient came complaining about pain on chewing on the tooth 3.7. Radiographically, a periapical radiolucency was clearly detectable. Retreatment was planned.

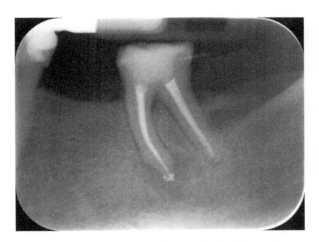

Figure 12.10 The tooth was filled with the BioConeless technique.

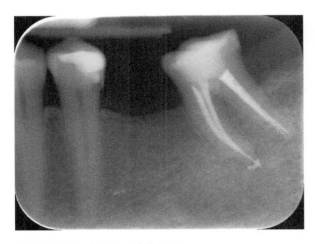

Figure 12.11 6 months follow-up.

the root canal apical to the stripping, without contaminating the stripping area that will be subsequently sealed with mineral trioxide aggregate (MTA) or bioceramic putty (Figures 12.12–12.15).

12.2.2 BioConeless: How to Do It?

The root canal system is shaped, cleaned, and adequately dried (Figure 12.16).

A small amount (2 mm in length) of bioceramic sealer (i.e. Brasseler, Savannah, GA, USA) is extruded from the syringe without the needle on a glass plate.

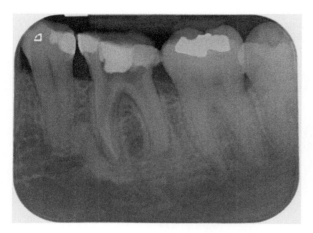

Figure 12.12 A patient was referred due to a iatrogenic error that led to the stripping of the mesial root of this first lower left molar.

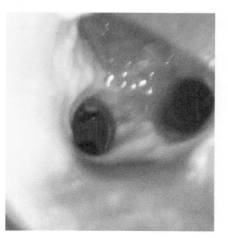

Figure 12.13 The clinical image shows the area of the stripping.

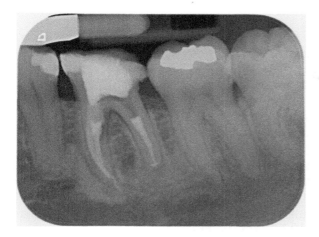

Figure 12.14 The tooth was filled with the sandwich technique, using BioConeless apical to the stripping in order to avoid any contamination of the area of communication between endodontium and periodontium.

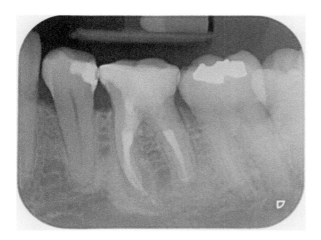

Figure 12.15 2 years follow-up.

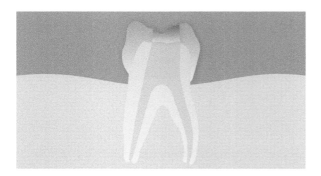

Figure 12.16 Root canals shaped and ready to be filled.

A plastic Thermafil carrier #20 (Dentsply Sirona, Ballaigues, Switzerland) is used to carry the bioceramic sealer into the canal, 1 mm short of the working length, with an up-and-down and rotation movement of the carrier (Figures 12.17–12.19). The placement is considered ideal when the tip of the carrier is completely covered by the sealer (Figure 12.19b). If the clinician is using a microscope during this phase, it will be possible to see that the root canal is completely covered by a thin film of sealer (Figure 12.20a–c).

The second step is to inject the gutta-percha with a dedicated injector (SuperEndo Beta, B&L Biotech, Gyeonggi-do, Korea) containing a new gutta-percha cylinder (Brasseler, Savannah, GA, USA) and equipped with a 23 G needle, set at the temperature of 200 °C. The needle is inserted into the root canal until stable, regardless of the distance from the apex (Figure 12.21). The stability of the needle is assessed exerting a gentle vibration on the gun, both mesiodistally and apically, in order to check that the needle is tightly in contact with the canal walls and will not be subjected to movements while extruding the gutta-percha.

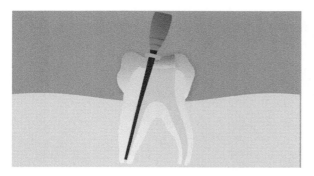

Figure 12.17 The Thermafil carrier arriving 1 mm short to the working length is chosen.

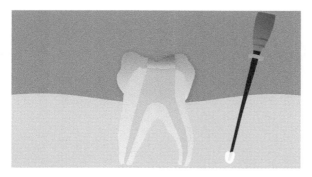

Figure 12.18 The bioceramic sealer is collected in a small amount from a glass slab.

(a)

(b)

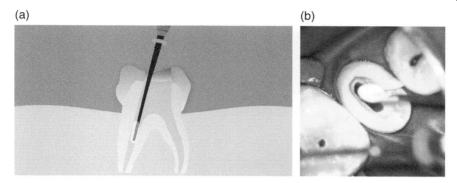

Figure 12.19 (a) The carrier is inserted into the root canal. (b) The tip of the carrier should be fully covered in sealer.

(a)

(b)

(c)

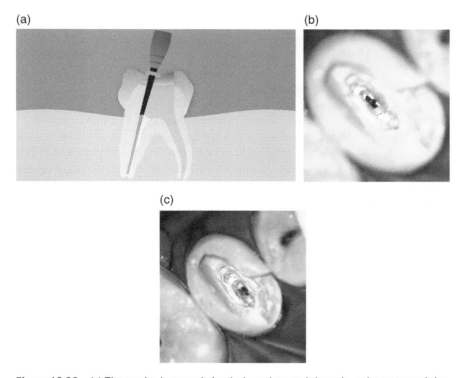

Figure 12.20 (a) The carrier is moved circularly and up and down in order to spread the sealer on the root canal walls. (b, c) The appearance the root canal should have after applying the sealer.

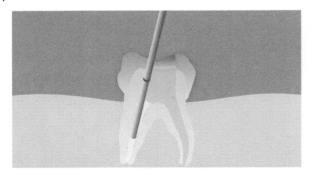

Figure 12.21   The gutta-percha injector is inserted into the root canal until finding a stable position.

The gutta percha is then slowly injected into the root canal, with a pull injection, until the operator feels a pushback. A mild resistance should then be applied on the gun in order to control the back-filling (Figures 12.22–12.26).

When the gutta-percha reaches the canal orifice, an adequate Schilder plugger is used to pack the soft gutta-percha into the canal (Figure 12.27).

It is advised to take an X-ray with the rubber dam to assess the adequacy of the obturation and, in case the filling is short, immediately remove the gutta-percha from the root canal and repeat.

The final step is to restore the tooth (Figure 12.28).

The principle that permits to fill the root canal is extremely close to that of the warm vertical compaction technique. The warm gutta-percha injected is compressed from one side by the pressure applied by the clinician's hand on the tip of the down-pack device and, on the other side, the apical constriction does not allow the gutta-percha to flow outside. This happens because the high amount of

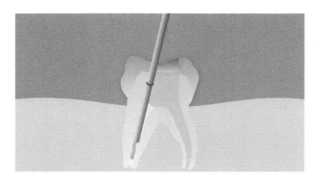

Figure 12.22   The needle is engaged and we start injecting gutta percha into the root canal with a constant and delicate pressure.

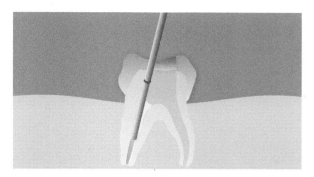

Figure 12.23 After six to seven seconds from the beginning of the extrusion, there is a push back sensation that has to be contrasted.

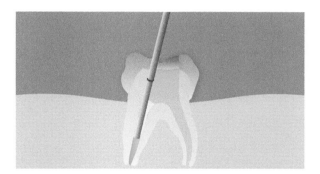

Figure 12.24 This is the most important moment of the technique: the taper of the preparation acts as a stop, the hand acts as coronal resistance and the gutta percha in packed into the apical third.

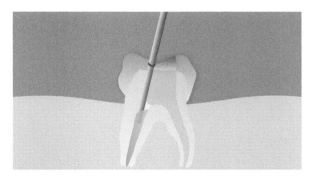

Figure 12.25 The extrusion of warm gutta-percha continues: the operator in this case has a different sensation because now the needle is not in contact with the walls of the root canal anymore.

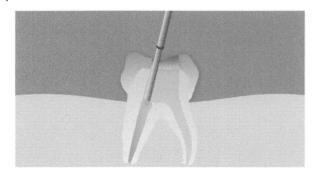

Figure 12.26 The root canal is filled up to the opening, preferably not over this limit.

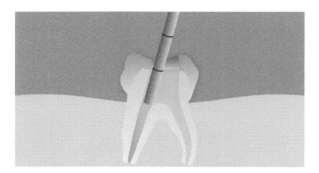

Figure 12.27 When the orifice is reached, the gutta-percha is packed with a plugger.

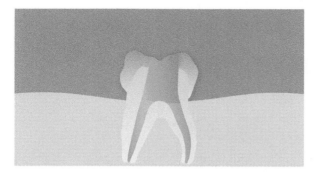

Figure 12.28 The tooth is restored.

gutta percha arriving to the apex starts cooling and the material tends to flow out coronally. If compared to the warm vertical compaction technique, this injection technique can be defined as warm vertical coneless technique or, briefly, Coneless®. When the Coneless is used with a bioceramic sealer, it is called BioConeless [36].

12.2.3 Concerns Regarding the Complete Filling of the Root Canal with the Coneless and BioConeless Techniques

The Coneless or BioConeless techniques are not particularly famous among clinicians. One of the main reasons for this is that most dentists are afraid to obtain an incorrect filling of the root canal system, with under- or overfilling.

In the BioConeless technique, underfilling might happen for a series of reasons such as:

1) Using a water-based sealer.
2) The tip of the back-fill device is not well fit into the root canal.
3) During the injection the patient feels pain and the operator moves the tip.
4) Being afraid of overfilling, the operator stops the procedure of injection of the warm gutta-percha before reaching the correct filling.

In these cases, it is advisable to immediately retreat the root canal before the sealer sets and to repeat the filling procedure.

The main concern regarding this technique was about its possible association with a high risk of extrusion of gutta-percha and sealer, possibly due to the lack of a pre-formed and calibrated gutta-percha cone to create a secure apical plug. Although Tennert et al. [37] have found impressive differences comparing the prevalence of material extrusion after carrier-based (Thermafil) and warm vertical compaction–based obturation techniques, but the extent of the extrusion was not recorded for comparison with other techniques. According to this article, the low risk of extrusion associated with the warm vertical compaction technique seems to be mainly ascribable to the fact that if the heat plugger is inserted at a safe distance from the apex (3–5 mm), the apical gutta-percha is not completely plasticized. No clinical study comparing the extrusion obtained with BioConeless and other techniques is available at the moment, but according to the clinical experience of the authors, the extrusion reported by Tennert is comparable to that observed with the BioConeless technique.

It should be noted that, regardless of the obturation technique, possible causes or factors favoring gutta-percha and/or sealer extrusion, such as canal transportation of the foramen due to over-instrumentation and apical deformation due to pre-existing apical periodontitis and incipient root resorption, persist.

As far as overfilling may be considered as an endodontic complication, Ricucci et al. [38] demonstrated that poor outcomes in treatment of teeth without signs of apical periodontitis were not associated with overfilling of the root canal. Apical periodontitis and postoperative symptoms in overfilled teeth seem to be strictly related to a coexisting infection, while they may not be ascribed to the cytotoxicity of the filling material. In fact, a variable inflammatory reaction usually develops in the periapical tissues contacting the filling materials, even when sealers remain within the canal space. Moreover, histological studies have shown that even though the inflammatory response to the extrusion of root filling materials in the apical periodontium may be severe in the short term, most sealers quickly lose their irritant components and become relatively inert. Additionally, most of the contemporary filling materials and sealers only exhibit significant cytotoxicity before setting [39]. Although the extraradicular presence of filling materials may not be held responsible for postendodontic disease, a considerable delay of the healing process may be found in some cases [40] (Figures 12.29–12.32).

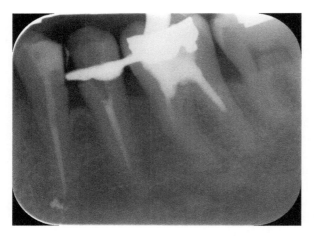

Figure 12.29 The patient referred the impossibility of chewing on the left side of the mouth. The X-ray revealed the presence of scarce endo-restorative treatments. The decision was to retreat teeth 3.5 and 3.6.

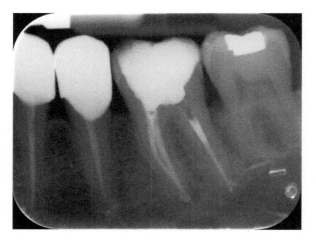

Figure 12.30 When retreating tooth 3.6, the Coneless technique was chosen to fill the root canal system. Some gutta-percha and sealer extrusion was noticed.

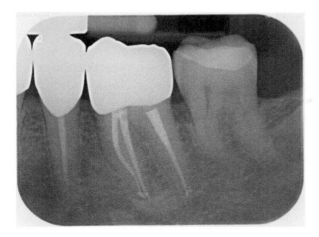

Figure 12.31 Despite the extrusion, the patient showed signs of healing at the follow-up and referred the complete disappearance of symptoms.

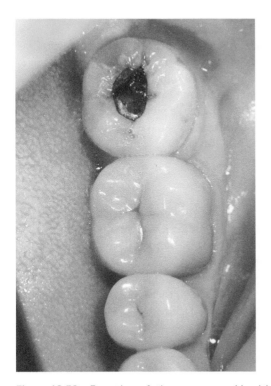

Figure 12.32 Even the soft tissues appeared healthy.

Li et al., in a study on 185 teeth filled with the single cone and bioceramic sealer technique, observed that in big lesions and large extrusions of bioceramic sealer, the healing rate was 96.8%. The difference in success rate of adequately filled teeth versus teeth with extrusion was not statistically significant. The article also stated that factors such as gender, age, tooth position, follow-up visit period, size of periapical lesion, treatment type, and extruding sealer amount had no influence on the outcome of the therapies [41].

12.2.4 Concerns Regarding the Consistency of the Obturation

Upon radiographic assessment, voids can be found in teeth filled with the BioConeless technique. These voids may be associated with air trapping inside the gun barrel, especially after replacement of the gutta-percha pellet. In fact, based on the Authors' feedback, a crackling sound could be heard each time a newly loaded gun was activated, and voids were found in the final X-ray. These voids can be fixed by heating the gutta percha with a heat carrier and packing it as in the warm vertical compaction technique.

12.2.4.1 Time Required to Complete the Obturation

The BioConeless protocol may provide the clinician with a time-saving workflow with respect to warm vertical condensation, especially because of the elimination of steps such as cone and plugger selection, pre-obturation X-ray, and gutta-percha compaction. With regard to carrier-based techniques, the Coneless protocol eliminates the need for carrier selection and cleaning of the pulp chamber, which is often necessary to eliminate the coronal part of the carrier when obturating multiple canals with such techniques and before restoration.

12.3 Final Remarks

In the Authors' experience, the BioConeless protocol for canal obturation has a minimal learning curve along with other several advantages. Among these, quality of the obturation upon radiographic assessment is satisfactory both in terms of extension and intracanal consistency. Moreover, lateral and accessory canals can be found and filled in a percentage that is close to the 27.4% presence of lateral and accessory canals found in a previous in vitro study.

One study by Bugea et al. considered the postoperative pain of teeth treated with several techniques, among which the BioConeless technique (injection of thermoplasticized gutta-percha with bioceramic sealer) was studied. The results were promising both in terms of postoperative pain and outcome [34].

The BioConeless technique can be particularly favorable when a fiber post restoration is needed after the endodontic treatment, as partial obturation of the root canal is easily obtained in order not to affect the adhesion during fiber post cementation and to provide an unaffected dentin substrate for hybridization. To reach this goal, the clinician has to remember that the preparation of the post space has to be done in the same appointment of the root canal filling in order to be sure that all the remnants of bioceramic sealer have been removed from the dentine of the root canal before the final setting of the material.

As opposed to warm vertical condensation, obturation by BioConeless technique can adapt to different tapers, as only a minimum taper is required for the plugger to reach 5 mm from the apex.

Lastly, relevant financial savings can be found, especially compared to carrier-based techniques, because the cost of the gutta-percha pellet is low and the amount of bioceramic sealer required to complete the obturation is minimal.

12.4   Learning Objectives

1) Know the filling technique that adapts the most to each case.
2) Learn to execute the BioConeless technique.
3) Know the indications and contraindications for the BioConeless technique.
4) Appreciate the advantages of the BioConeless technique in terms of ergonomics.

References

1 Schilder, H. (1967). Filling root canals in three dimensions. *Dental Clinics of North America* 723: 723–744.

2 Baser Can, E.D., Keles, A., and Aslan, B. (2017). Micro-CT evaluation of the quality of root fillings when using three root filling systems. *International Endodontic Journal* 50 (5): 499–505.

3 Bhandi, S., Mashyakhy, M., Abumelha, A.S. et al. (2021). Complete obturation-cold lateral condensation vs. thermoplastic techniques: a systematic review of micro-CT studies. *Materials (Basel).* 14 (14).

4 Xu, Q., Ling, J., Cheung, G.S., and Hu, Y. (2007). A quantitative evaluation of sealing ability of 4 obturation techniques by using a glucose leakage test. *Oral Surgery, Oral Medicine, Oral Pathology, Oral Radiology, and Endodontics* 104: e109–e113.

5 Wu, M.K., Kastakova, A., and Wesselink, P.R. (2001). Quality of cold and warm gutta-percha fillings in oval canals in mandibular premolars. *International Endodontic Journal* 34: 485–491.

6 Dasari, L., Anwarullah, A., Mandava, J. et al. (2020). Influence of obturation technique on penetration depth and adaptation of a bioceramic root canal sealer. *Journal of conservative dentistry: JCD.* 23 (5): 505–511.

7 Akhtar, H., Naz, F., Hasan, A. et al. (2023). Exploring the most effective apical seal for contemporary bioceramic and conventional endodontic sealers using three obturation techniques. *Medicina (Kaunas)* 59 (3): 567. https://doi.org/10.3390/medicina59030567.

8 Collins, J., Walker, M.P., Kulild, J., and Lee, C. (2006). A comparison of three gutta-percha obturation techniques to replicate canal irregularities. *Journal of Endodontia* 32: 762–765.

9 Yee, F.S., Marlin, J., Krakow, A.A., and Gron, P. (1977). Three-dimensional obturation of the root canal using injection-molded, thermoplasticized dental gutta-percha. *Journal of Endodontia* 3 (5): 168–174.

10 Marlin, J., Krakow, A.A., Desilets, R.P. Jr., and Gron, P. (1981). Clinical use of injection-molded thermoplasticized gutta-percha for obturation of the root canal system: a preliminary report. *Journal of Endodontia* 7 (6): 277–281.

11 Torabinejad, M., Skobe, Z., Trombly, P.L. et al. (1978). Scanning electron microscopic study of root canal obturation using thermoplasticized gutta-percha. *Journal of Endodontia* 4 (8): 245–250.

12 Michanowicz, A.E., Michanowicz, J.P., Michanowicz, A.M. et al. (1989). Clinical evaluation of low-temperature thermoplasticized injectable gutta-percha: a preliminary report. *Journal of Endodontia* 15 (12): 602–607.

13 De Angelis, F., D'Arcangelo, C., Buonvivere, M. et al. (2021). In vitro microleakage evaluation of bioceramic and zinc-eugenol sealers with two obturation techniques. *Coatings* 11 (6): 727.

14 Sobarzo-Navarro, V. (1991). Clinical experience in root canal obturation by an injection thermoplasticized gutta-percha technique. *Journal of Endodontia* 17 (8): 389–391.

15 Castellucci, A. and Gambarini, G. (1995). Obturation of iatrogenically damaged root canals with injectable thermoplasticized gutta-percha: a case report. *International Endodontic Journal* 28 (2): 108–110.

16 Abdellatif, D., Amato, A., Calapaj, M. et al. (2021). A novel modified obturation technique using biosealers: an ex vivo study. *Journal of Conservative Dentistry* 24 (4): 369–373.

17 Pontoriero, D.I.K., Madaro, G., Vanagolli, V. et al. (2021). Sealing ability of a bioceramic sealer used in combination with cold and warm obturation techniques. *Journal of Osseointegration* 13 (4): 248–255.

18 Stropko, J.J. (2008). The system "S" technique: to seal the entire canal system for "success". *Roots.* 4: 6–18.

19 Kumar, N.S., Prabu, P.S., Prabu, N., and Rathinasamy, S. (2012). Sealing ability of lateral condensation, thermoplasticized gutta-percha and flowable gutta-percha obturation techniques: a comparative in vitro study. *Journal of Pharmacy & Bioallied Sciences* 4 (Suppl 2): S131–S135.

20 Zhang, W., Li, Z., and Peng, B. (2009). Assessment of a new root canal sealer's apical sealing ability. *Oral Surgery, Oral Medicine, Oral Pathology, Oral Radiology, and Endodontics* 107 (6): e79–e82.

21 Parirokh, M. and Torabinejad, M. (2010). Mineral trioxide aggregate: a comprehensive literature review--part III: clinical applications, drawbacks, and mechanism of action. *Journal of Endodontia* 36 (3): 400–413.

22 Chybowski, E.A., Glickman, G.N., Patel, Y. et al. (2018). Clinical outcome of non-surgical root canal treatment using a single-cone technique with endosequence bioceramic sealer: a retrospective analysis. *Journal of Endodontia* 44 (6): 941–945.

23 Bardini, G., Casula, L., Ambu, E. et al. (2021). A 12-month follow-up of primary and secondary root canal treatment in teeth obturated with a hydraulic sealer. *Clinical Oral Investigations* 25 (5): 2757–2764.

24 Drukteinis, S. and Camilleri, J. (2021). *Bioceramic Materials in Clinical Endodontics*, 101. Springer.

25 Keles, A., Alcin, H., Kamalak, A., and Versiani, M.A. (2014). Micro-CT evaluation of root filling quality in oval-shaped canals. *International Endodontic Journal* 47 (12): 1177–1184.

26 Celikten, B., Uzuntas, C.F., Orhan, A.I. et al. (2016). Evaluation of root canal sealer filling quality using a single-cone technique in oval shaped canals: an in vitro Micro-CT study. *Scanning* 38: 133–140.

27 Penha da Silva, P.J., Marceliano-Alves, M.F., Provenzano, J.C. et al. (2021). Quality of root canal filling using a bioceramic sealer in oval canals: a three-dimensional analysis. *European Journal of Dentistry.* July (3): 475–480.

28 Wu, M.K. and Wesselink, P.R. (2001). A primary observation on the preparation and obturation of oval canals. *International Endodontic Journal* 34 (2): 137–141.

29 Jarrett, I.S., Marx, D., Covey, D. et al. (2004). Percentage of canals filled in apical cross sections – an in vitro study of seven obturation techniques. *International Endodontic Journal* 37: 392–398.

30 Versiani, M.A., Pecora, J.D., and de Sousa-Neto, M.D. (2011). Flat-oval root canal preparation with self-adjusting file instrument: a micro-computed tomography study. *Journal of Endodontia* 37 (7): 1002–1007.

31 Siqueira, J.F. Jr., Perez, A.R., Marceliano-Alves, M.F. et al. (2018). What happens to unprepared root canal walls: a correlative analysis using micro-computed tomography and histology/scanning electron microscopy. *International Endodontic Journal* 51 (5): 501–508.

32 Torabinejad, M., Ung, B., and Kettering, J.D. (1990). In vitro bacterial penetration of coronally unsealed endodontically treated teeth. *Journal of Endodontia* 16 (12): 566–569.

33 Chen, B., Haapasalo, M., Mobuchon, C. et al. (2020). Cytotoxicity and the effect of temperature on physical properties and chemical composition of a new calcium silicate-based root canal sealer. *Journal of Endodontia* 46 (4): 531–538.

34 Bugea, C., Cerutti, F., Ongaro, F. et al. (2022). Postoperative pain and one year follow up success rate of warm vertical compaction, single cone, coneless and bioconeless obturation methods. *Journal of Osseointegration.* 14 (4): 209–216.

35 Budd, C.S., Weller, R.N., and Kulild, J.C. (1991). A comparison of thermoplasticized injectable gutta-percha obturation techniques. *Journal of Endodontia* 17 (6): 260–264.

36 Bugea, C., Pontoriero, D.I.K., Rosenberg, G. et al. (2022). Maxillary premolars with four canals: case series. *Bioengineering* 9: 757.

37 Tennert, C., Jungbäck, I.L., and Wrbas, K.T. (2013). Comparison between two thermoplastic root canal obturation techniques regarding extrusion of root canal filling--a retrospective in vivo study. *Clinical Oral Investigations* 17 (2): 449–454.

38 Ricucci, D., Rôças, I.N., Alves, F.R. et al. (2016). Apically extruded sealers: fate and influence on treatment outcome. *Journal of Endodontia* 42 (2): 243–249.

39 Komabayashi, T., Colmenar, D., Cvach, N. et al. (2020). Comprehensive review of current endodontic sealers. *Dental Materials* 39 (5): 703–720.

40 Aminoshariae, A. and Kulild, J.C. (2020). The impact of sealer extrusion on endodontic outcome: a systematic review with meta-analysis. *Australian Endodontic Journal: The Journal of the Australian Society of Endodontology Inc.* 46 (1): 123–129. https://doi.org/10.1111/aej.12370.

41 Li, J., Chen, L., Zeng, C. et al. (2022). Clinical outcome of bioceramic sealer iRoot SP extrusion in root canal treatment: a retrospective analysis. *Head & Face Medicine* 31 (1): 28.

13

Primary Endodontic Treatment using ProTaper Ultimate and AH Plus Bioceramic Sealer

Viresh Chopra[1,2,3] and Harneet Chopra[1]

[1] *Adult Restorative Dentistry, Oman Dental College, Muscat, Oman*
[2] *Endodontology, Oman Dental College, Muscat, Oman*
[3] *Bart's London School of Medicine and Dentistry, Queen Mary University, London, UK*

13.1 Introduction of the Case

Case of upper right maxillary first molar with porcelain fused to metal crown.

13.1.1 Patient Information

- Age:32
- Gender: Male
- Medical history: Noncontributory

13.1.2 Tooth

- **Identification**: Right maxillary first molar (Tooth 16)
- **Dental history**:
  Chief complaint: Patient reported with a chief complaint of tenderness on biting. Occasionally, he felt sensitivity to hot and cold. In addition, complaints of bad taste occasionally.
- **Clinical examination findings**:
  Tooth 16 is tender to percussion and had a porcelain fused to metal (PFM) crown. The crown was attached to another PFM crown on 15.
- **Preoperative radiological assessment**:
  The periapical radiograph revealed previous root canal treatment in 15. The following are the observations after reading the preoperative radiograph: (Figure 13.1)
- Short obturation in all the canals.
- Periapical radiolucency around the root of 15
- Suspected fractured instrument in the apical part of the palatal root.

The patient was made aware of the inadequate RCT in relation to 15, but he wanted to treat only the symptomatic tooth, which was 16 in this case. It was made clear to the patient that the investigations can be concluded only after removing the crowns where it will be possible to perform sensibility testing. Once the crowns were removed sensibility testing was performed where the tooth showed delayed response on electric pulp testing (EPT) and only the palatal surface responded to cold testing. The tooth did not respond to heat test at all.

- **Diagnosis** (pulpal and periapical): Partially necrotic teeth with symptomatic apical periodontitis.

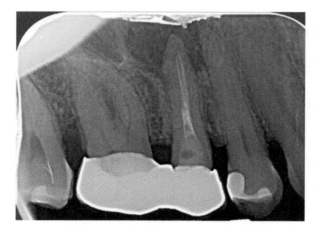

Figure 13.1 Preoperative radiograph.

Root canal treatment of teeth Federation Dentaire Internationale (FDI) 16 and retreatment of 15 was advised to the patient. However, patient wanted to treat only tooth 16. The patient was informed about future course of the lesion (infection) in 15 and what it can lead to.

- **Treatment plan**

The treatment was planned in different stages:

Stage 1:
- Local anesthetic administration
- Rubber dam isolation
- Gaining entry in the pulp chamber and locating orifices
- Locating the canals
- Exploring the access cavity for extra canals
- Orifice widening

Stage 2:
- Establishing a glide path
- Working length determination (electronic and radiographic)
- Orifice widening
- Cleaning and shaping as per the rotary protocol

Stage 3:
- Master cone verification
- 3D obturation using bioceramic sealer and gutta-percha (GP)
- Core buildup

Disinfection with irrigants was carried on throughout the root canal procedure as per the recommended protocol.

13.2 Treatment Procedure for the First Appointment

Superior alveolar nerve block and palatine block anesthesia was administered and the tooth was isolated with rubber dam isolation (Figure 13.2). The leakage spaces were isolated with liquid rubber dam. The treatment was initiated under a microscope. Occlusal surface showed resin composite restoration along with remaining residual caries (Figure 13.2).

The first step was to make an endodontic access cavity and then look for the dentinal map. The map will guide us to the orifices (Figure 13.3). Endodontic ultrasonic tips were used to modify the access cavity and adhere to the guidelines of minimal invasive endodontics. Once the access cavity was prepared to have a straight line access to the canals, orifice widening was done using orifice widener rotary file (Dentsply Sirona, USA) (Video 13.1).

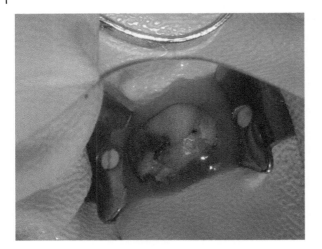

Figure 13.2 Rubber dam isolation.

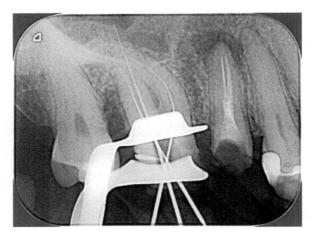

Figure 13.3 PA radiograph to verify the electronic working length.

Following orifice widening, glide path to the canals was established using 10K hand files. Intracanal medicament was placed and the patient was recalled for the next appointment for working length determination and completion of root canal treatment.

13.3 Treatment Procedure for the Second Appointment

The second appointment was planned to continue the root canal treatment following working length determination, cleaning, and shaping and obturation.

Once the full working length was achieved electronically, periapical radiograph was taken to confirm the same (Figure 13.3).

The canals were finally cleaned and shaped with ProTaper Ultimate files up to size 25/04. EDTA gel, saline, 2.5% sodium hypochlorite, and EDTA liquid were used as irrigants alternatively. Irrigation was done using TruNatomy needles (Dentsply Sirona, USA). Ultrasonic agitation of the irrigants was done with EndoUltra from Dentsply (Video 13.2).

Clinically, the fit of the master cones was checked and verified with a periapical radiograph at the calculated working length (Figure 13.4).

Once the master cone fit was confirmed, the canals were left moist and excessive moisture removed with the help of paper points. The premixed injectable AH Plus Bioceramic sealer (Dentsply Sirona, USA) was applied inside the canals and the master cones were coated with the sealer and placed inside the canals. The gutta-percha was cut at the orifice level with heated plugger (Video 13.3). All the canals were obturated with warm vertical condensation technique and the pulp chamber cleaned of any gutta-percha or sealer (Video 13.4). Immediate postoperative radiograph was taken to verify the final obturation (Figure 13.5).

Figure 13.4 PA radiograph to verify the length/fit of master cones.

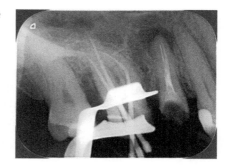

Figure 13.5 PA radiograph immediately after obturation.

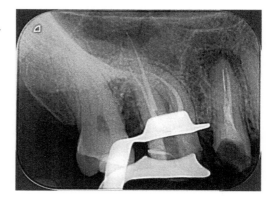

13.3.1 Irrigation Protocol

- Hand files were used with EDTA gel, rinsing with saline.
- TruNatomy irrigation needles were used.
- 2.5% sodium hypochlorite throughout the cleaning and shaping procedure. Rinsed with saline.
- 17% EDTA 1 ml/canal with sonic/ultrasonic activation. Rinsed with saline.
- Final rinse with 2.5% sodium hypochlorite with internal heating with any instrument, e.g. Touch 'n Heat, and sonic ultrasonic activation for 20–30 seconds per canal.

Flushing with saline between irrigants is must as it will stop the irrigants from reacting with each other.

Materials used for obturation: Premixed injectable AH Plus Bioceramic root canal sealer, ProTaper Ultimate gutta-perchas.

13.4 Technical Aspects

Root canal treatment protocol has evolved with time. With the advent of time, more advanced cleaning and shaping instruments have been developed. These NiTi instruments focus on anatomical shaping while adhering to the guidelines of minimal invasive endodontics. Endodontic ultrasonic tips should be used to stay conservative while cutting tooth structure and modifying access cavities. Excessive removal of tooth structure might lead to fracture of the tooth due to low strength. Copious irrigation should be maintained throughout the procedure. Care should be taken not to ever use the endodontic files in dry canals.

13.4.1 Follow up

Patient became asymptomatic after the root canal treatment.

13.5 Learning Objectives

The reader should be able to understand the following.

- The significance of proper reading of the preoperative radiograph.
- The importance of using endodontic ultrasonic tips to modify the endodontic access cavity.
- Emphasis on achieving straight line access cannot be ignored.
- The role of irrigants for disinfecting the root canal system.

- Using flexible TruNatomy irrigation needles helps the needle to adapt to the shape and curvature of the root canal.
- The importance of incorporating the whole root canal system in the disinfection process during primary root canal treatment.
- How to decide clinically which instrument is to be used for a particular step during an primary endodontic treatment.
- The importance of using the right materials to initiate body healing.
- The concepts of understanding the prognosis of the tooth and trying to save the tooth instead of straight away extracting it.

To access the videos for this chapter, please go to

www.wiley.com/go/chopra/bioceramicsinendodontics

VIDEO 13.1 Orifice widening.
VIDEO 13.2 Cleaning and shaping.
VIDEO 13.3 Sealer application and obturation.
VIDEO 13.4 Obturation in all canals.

14

Management of Failed Root Canal Treatment in an Anterior Tooth Using Calcium Silicate Cement

Viresh Chopra[1,2,3] *and Ajinkya Pawar*[4]

[1] *Adult Restorative Dentistry, Oman Dental College, Muscat, Oman*
[2] *Endodontology, Oman Dental College, Muscat, Oman*
[3] *Bart's London School of Medicine and Dentistry, Queen Mary University, London, UK*
[4] *Conservative Dentistry and Endodontics, Nair Hospital Dental College, Mumbai, India*

CONTENTS

14.1 Introduction of the Case

Case of failed root canal treatment associated with a previous inadequate root canal treatment and suspected inadequate obturation. The patient reported with symptomatic apical periodontitis (SAP).

Bioceramics in Endodontics, First Edition. Edited by Viresh Chopra.
© 2024 John Wiley & Sons, Inc. Published 2024 by John Wiley & Sons, Inc.
Companion website: www.wiley.com/go/chopra/bioceramicsinendodontics

14.1.1 Patient Information

- Age: 28
- Gender: Female
- Medical history: Noncontributory
- Identification of the tooth: Right maxillary central incisor (Tooth 11)
- **Dental history**:

  Chief complaint: Patient reported with a chief complaint of tenderness on biting. Occasionally, she felt swelling between teeth 11 and 12. The buccal vestibule between 11 and 12 is tender to touch.

  - **Clinical examination findings:**

    The tooth 11 is tender to percussion.

  - **Preoperative radiological assessment**:

    The periapical radiograph revealed previous root canal treatment in 11. The following are the observations after reading the preoperative radiograph: (Figure 14.1)

  - Inadequate obturation with suspected poor lateral condensation.
  - Periapical radiolucency around the root of 11

The patient was made aware of the inadequate RCT in relation to 11 and advised her to re-treat the same tooth nonsurgically (NSRCT).

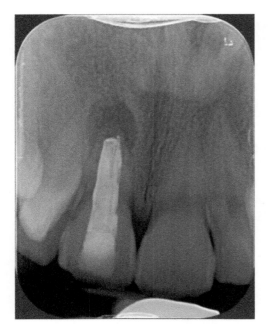

Figure 14.1 Preoperative radiograph.

14.1.2 Diagnosis (Pulpal and Periapical)

Failed primary root canal treatment with SAP.

14.1.2.1 Advice
Nonsurgical re-treatment of 11 was advised to the patient. The patient agreed for the treatment.

14.2 Treatment Plan

The treatment was planned in different stages:

Stage 1:
- Local anesthetic administration
- Rubber dam isolation
- Gaining entry in the canal and locating previous gutta-percha (GP)
- Removal of previous GP
- Placement of intracanal medicament (IM)

Stage 2:
- Removal of IM
- Working length determination (electronic and radiographic)
- Cleaning and disinfection
- Placement of calcium silicate cement.

Stage 3:
- Obturation with thermoplasticized GP
- Core buildup

14.2.1 Treatment Procedure for the First Appointment

Buccal infiltration anesthesia was administered and rubber dam placed for isolation. The endodontic access was gained using Endo-Z bur. Resin composite restoration was removed to reveal the previous GP in the canal. Once located, the previous GP was removed using endo shaper files (FKG Dentaire, Switzerland). Once the GP was completely removed periapical (PA) radiograph was taken to verify the same (Figure 14.2).

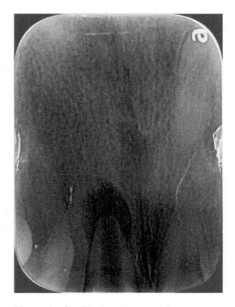

Figure 14.2 PA showing complete removal of GP.

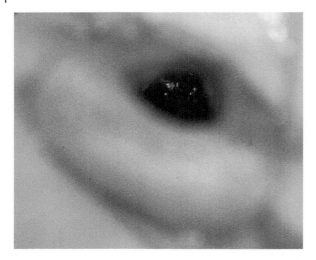

Figure 14.3 Wide open apex clearly visible under magnification.

The apex was clearly visualized under the microscope (OPMI Pico, Carl Zeiss, Germany) (Figure 14.3).

IM (Opacal, Produits Dentaires, SA) was used between the appointments. It was injected with dispensing syringe directly inside the canal (Video 14.1). The patient was recalled for completion of root canal retreatment.

14.2.2 Treatment Procedure for the Second Appointment

The second appointment was planned to continue the root canal retreatment with adequate disinfection followed with apical plug formation with calcium silicate cement. Mineral trioxide aggregate (MTA) (Produits Dentaires, Switzerland) was used as an apical plug material.

The estimated length of MTA placement was measured by placing a plugger that goes to 2 mm short of the established working length.

MTA was placed using micro apical plug system (MAP system) (Produits Dentaires, Switzerland). Incremental placement followed by gentle condensation was done in order to create an adequate apical plug (Video 14.2). Once the apical plug was formed, it was verified clinically as well as radiographically (Figures 14.4 and 14.5).

Following apical plug formation with MTA, the canal was obturated with thermoplasticized GP using Fast Pack and Fast Fill (Eighteeth, China) (Video 14.3h).

The obturation was verified clinically as well as with an immediate post-obturation radiograph (Figures 14.6 and 14.7).

Figure 14.4 Clinical verification of MTA under DOM.

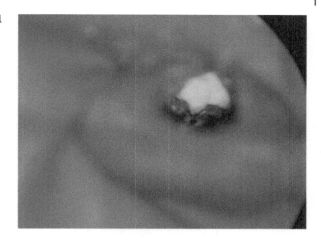

Figure 14.5 Radiographic verification of apical barrier placement.

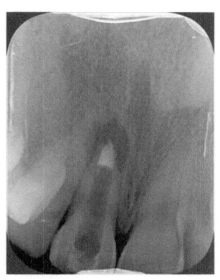

Figure 14.6 Obturation of the root canal using thermoplasticized GP.

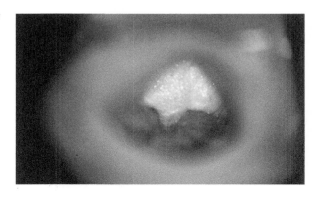

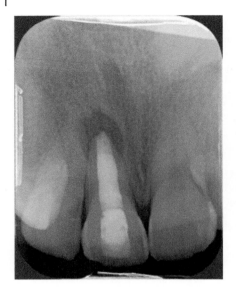

Figure 14.7 PA radiograph to verify the obturation.

14.2.3 Irrigation Protocol

- Hand files were used with EDTA gel, rinsing with saline.
- TruNatomy irrigation needles were used.
- 2.5% sodium hypochlorite throughout the cleaning and shaping procedure. Rinse with saline.
- 17% EDTA 1ml/canal with sonic/ultrasonic activation. Rinse with saline.
- Final rinse with 2.5% sodium hypochlorite with internal heating with any instrument, e.g. Touch'n Heat, and sonic ultrasonic activation for 20–30 seconds per canal.

Flushing with saline between irrigants is a must, as it will stop the irrigants from reacting with each other.

14.2.3.1 Materials Used for Obturation

Calcium silicate cement as apical plug barrier, thermoplasticized GP as core obturation material.

14.3 Technical Aspects

Root canal retreatment required certain specific case related considerations in order to achieve success. The first and foremost is complete removal of previous GP. Adequate instruments should be used to ensure that the canal is free of any residual filling material. The second consideration in such a case is that it requires minimal shaping but more of disinfection. However, care needs to be taken that the irrigant (sodium hypochlorite) should not go in the periapical area, else sodium hypochlorite accident can happen.

The third consideration is to calculate the exact area/length where MTA needs to be placed. MTA being a very biocompatible material is very friendly beyond the periapical area. However, it is not required in the periapical area, therefore, an attempt should be made to place it right at the apex. Cone beam computed tomography (CBCT) is of prime importance in such a case. However, patient could not afford it, therefore, we had to perform re-treatment without CBCT.

Lastly, choosing the correct obturation technique is an important factor in deciding the success of the treatment provided.

14.3.1 Follow-up

Patient became asymptomatic after the root canal treatment and follow-up radiographs show periapical healing.

14.4 Learning Objectives

The reader should be able to understand the following:

- The significance of proper reading of the preoperative radiograph.
- The emphasis on achieving straight line access cannot be ignored.
- The role of irrigants for disinfecting the root canal system.
- The role of using adequate files to remove GP from the root canals.
- The importance of incorporating the whole root canal system in the disinfection process during primary root canal treatment.
- Choosing the correct material for apical plug barrier.
- Placement of apical barrier material with adequate tools such as MAP system.
- Choosing the correct obturation technique.

 To access the videos for this chapter, please go to

www.wiley.com/go/chopra/bioceramicsinendodontics

VIDEO 14.1   Placement of intracanal medicament.
VIDEO 14.2   Placement of MTA.
VIDEO 14.3h   Placement of thermoplasticised GP.

15

Apexification of a Traumatic Central Incisor with an Apical Plug Technique using Calcium Silicate Cement

Viresh Chopra[1,2,3], Harneet Chopra[1], and Aylin Baysan[3]

[1] *Adult Restorative Dentistry, Oman Dental College, Muscat, Oman*
[2] *Endodontology, Oman Dental College, Muscat, Oman*
[3] *Bart's London School of Medicine and Dentistry, Queen Mary University, London, UK*

CONTENTS

Bioceramics in Endodontics, First Edition. Edited by Viresh Chopra.
© 2024 John Wiley & Sons, Inc. Published 2024 by John Wiley & Sons, Inc.
Companion website: www.wiley.com/go/chopra/bioceramicsinendodontics

15.1 Introduction of the Case

Case of management of a wide open apex traumatic upper right maxillary central incisor associated with periapical radiolucency.

15.1.1 Patient Information

- Age: 20
- Gender: Male
- Medical history: Noncontributory

15.1.2 Tooth Information

15.1.2.1 Identification
Right maxillary central incisor (Tooth 11)

15.1.2.2 Dental History
Chief complaint: Patient reported with a chief complaint of intraoral swelling with tenderness on biting.

15.1.2.3 Clinical Examination Findings
Tooth 11 was tender to percussion. The buccal vestibule had intraoral swelling with tenderness on palpation.

Investigations
Preoperative radiological assessment:
 The periapical radiograph revealed periapical radiolucency in relation to (irt) #11. The tooth had a wide open apex (Figure 15.1).

Sensibility Testing
1) Hot and cold test: No response
2) Electric pulp test (EPT): No response
3) Tenderness to percussion: Positive

15.1.2.4 Diagnosis (Pulpal and Periapical)
Necrotic pulp with symptomatic apical periodontitis (SAP)

15.1.2.5 Advice
Root canal treatment with apical plug formation (apexification) using calcium silicate cement followed by obturation of the remaining root canal space

15.2 Treatment Plan

The treatment was planned in different stages:

Figure 15.1 Preoperative periapical radiograph showing wide open apex with periapical radiolucency.

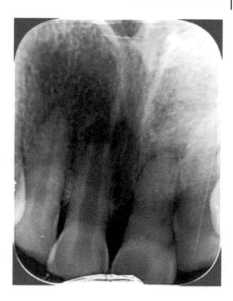

Stage 1
- Gaining entry in the pulp chamber and locating the orifice
- Irrigating the canal
- Cleaning and disinfection of the root canal system
- Placement of intracanal medicament

Stage 2
- Removal of intracanal medicament
- Cleaning and shaping the canals (more of disinfection and less of shaping)
- Placement of calcium silicate cement amd formation of apical plug

Stage 3
- Obturation of the remainder root canal space using thermoplasticized GP
- Core buildup with resin composite
- Postenedodontic full coverage restoration

15.2.1 Treatment Procedure for the First Appointment

Buccal infiltration anesthesia was administered and the tooth was isolated with rubber dam isolation. The endodontic access cavity was initiated under dental operating microscope (DOM). Once the canal was located, it was irrigated with 3% sodium hypochlorite using IrriFlex (Produits Dentaires, Switzerland). The irrigation needle was chosen due to its flexible design and side vented portal of exits.

The canal was already wide, therefore minimal shaping was decided for this case.The canal was filled with the irrigant and cleaned and shaped with Endoshaper file (FKG Dentaire, Switzerland). This file was chosen due to its three-dimensional design which can throw the irrigant in every corner of the canal, thus helping in adequate disnfection along with minimal shaping. Intracanl medicament was placed and patient recalled after one week.

15.2.2 Treatment Procedure for the Second Appointment

The second appointment was planned to remove the intracanal medicament and attempt to observe the wide open apex which had blood. (Figure 15.2)

The canal was made dry with paper points and the working length reconfirmed with suitable size endodontic plugger. The plugger was used in order to decide the length which will be 2-3 mm short of the working length where plugger can condense the apical plug. (Figure 15.3)

Once the length was confirmed, the canal was prepared to receive the calcium silicate cement, Mineral trioxide aggregate (MTA) in this case. Manipulation of MTA was done per the manufacturer's instructions and micro apical plug, i.e. MAP system (Produits Dentaires, Switzerland), was chosen to be used as a carrier to carry MTA up to the open apex (Video 15.1).

Immediate postoperative radiograph was taken to check the extension of the apical plug (Figure 15.4).

Temporary dressing was provided and the patient was recalled for obturation of the remaining root canal space.

15.2.3 Treatment Procedure for the Third Appointment

The patient was asymptomatic and it was decided to move ahead with the treatment plan. The decision to obturate the canal with thermoplasticized gutta-percha (GP)

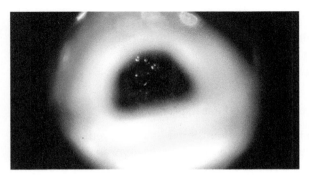

Figure 15.2 Wide open apex under dental operating microscope.

using Fast Fill and Fast Pack systems (Eighteeth, China) was made. The root canal space was filled with increments of melted GP with subsequent condensation with a suitable endodontic plugger (Video 15.2). The final obturation was seen clinically (Figure 15.5) as well as radiographically (Figure 15.6).

Core buildup was done using resin composite and the patient was recalled for post endodontic full coverage restoration.

15.2.3.1 Irrigation Protocol

- 2.5% sodium hypochlorite throughout the cleaning and shaping procedure. Rinse with saline.
- 17% EDTA 1 ml/canal with sonic/ultrasonic activation. Rinse with saline.
- Final rinse with 2.5% sodium hypochlorite with internal heating with any instrument, e.g. Touch'n Heat, and sonic ultrasonic activation for 20–30 seconds per canal.

Flushing with saline between irrigants is a must, as it will stop the irrigants from reacting with each other.

Materials used for obturation: MTA for apical plug, thermoplasticized GP for obturation, resin composite for core buildup.

15.3 Technical Aspects

Traumatic injuries during tooth development can lead to failure in complete root development. In such cases, the root fails to achieve a natural constriction and we often see wide open apices

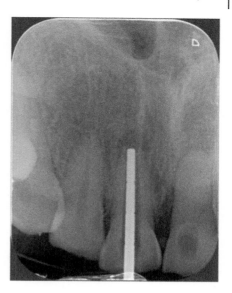

Figure 15.3 PA radiograph with endodontic plugger.

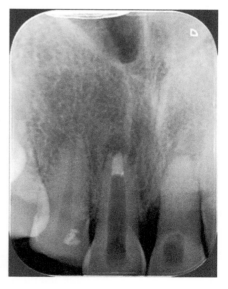

Figure 15.4 Apical plug formation.

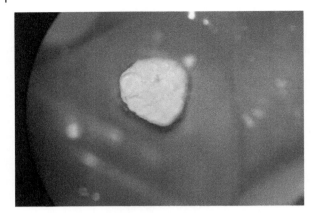

Figure 15.5   Final obturation with thermoplasticised GP.

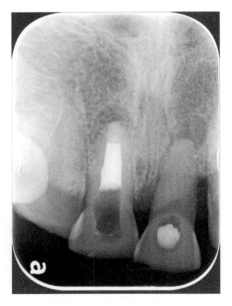

Figure 15.6   PA radiograph immediately after obturation.

accoumpanied with necrotic pulps. This is generally detected when the patient visits the dentist due to feeling tenderness on eating or intraoral swelling or sinus discharge in relation to those teeth. Wide open apex is observed in the PA. It is the result of the traumatic injury few years back. Regeneration can be an option but for that health periapical tissues are required.

In such cases where apexification is the treatment of choice, the following care should be taken:

- Minimal shaping of the root canals
- Maximum disinfection with recommended irrigation protocol
- Not pushing the irrigant beyond the apex in the periapical area
- Measure the extent to which endodontic plugger should go
- Placement of MTA at an adequate length
- Do not use excessive force and push MTA in the periapical area
- Once MTA is set, fill the root canal space with thermoplasticized GP technique with gentle condensation.

Copious irrigation should be maintained throughout the procedure and endodontic files should not be used in dry canals.

15.3.1 Follow-up

A six-month followup radiograph shows significant healing of the periradicular area (Figure 15.7).

15.4 Learning Objectives

The reader should be able to understand the following:

- The significance of proper reading of the preoperative radiograph.
- Relate the radiographic findings with dental history of the patient.
- The treatment plan to manage wide open apex cases.
- The significance of sensibility testing to reach a proper diagnosis.
- The role of irrigants for disinfecting the root canal system.
- The choice of correct shaping technique in cases with weak root canal walls.
- How to choose the correct material for apical plug formation.
- The technique, armamentarium required for apical plug formation.
- The technique needed for filling the root canal space.
- The concepts of understanding the prognosis of the tooth and trying to save the tooth instead of straight away extracting it.

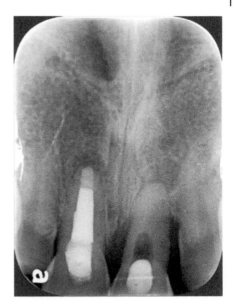

Figure 15.7 PA radiograph after core buildup.

15.5 Conclusion

Traumatic anterior teeth with wide open apex can be suitably managed with regeneration or apexification owing to the indications by the tooth and periapical areas.

To access the videos for this chapter, please go to

www.wiley.com/go/chopra/bioceramicsinendodontics

VIDEO 15.1 Apical plug formation using MTA.
VIDEO 15.2 Obturation of root canal space using thermoplasticised GP.

16

Coneless Obturations: Bioceramics as Obturating Materials

Viresh Chopra[1,2,3] and Maryam Hasnain[4]

[1] Endodontology, Oman Dental College, Muscat, Oman
[2] Adult Restorative Dentistry, Oman Dental College, Muscat, Oman
[3] Bart's London School of Medicine and Dentistry, Queen Mary University, London, UK
[4] Private Practitioner, Birmingham, UK

CONTENTS

Bioceramics in Endodontics, First Edition. Edited by Viresh Chopra.
© 2024 John Wiley & Sons, Inc. Published 2024 by John Wiley & Sons, Inc.
Companion website: www.wiley.com/go/chopra/bioceramicsinendodontics

16.1   Introduction

Root canal filling materials are used when the inside of a tooth (called the pulp) is damaged or infected and needs to be cleaned out. This usually happens when the pulp is hurt by an injury, cavities, or dental work. Removing the damaged pulp helps to save the tooth. Sometimes, dentists may also remove the pulp on purpose to use the space for other dental treatments [1].

There are two ways to fill root canals depending on the root's development: apexification for immature roots and root canal obturation for fully developed roots. Traditional methods have evolved in the last 20 years due to new dental materials like Mineral Trioxide Aggregate (MTA) and Bioceramics. These materials were created to resist deterioration when in contact with moisture, improving their properties for better treatment outcomes. Initially, MTA was introduced as root end filling material and for root perforation repairs. Its use also extended as root canal sealer and apexification material [2]. However, MTA had few clinical concerns such as discoloration [3], longer setting time [4], and consistency of freshly mixed material [1]. To solve problems linked to trace elements and aluminum in dental materials, second-generation materials switched to using pure tricalcium silicate cement instead of Portland cement.

In traditional root canal treatment for mature teeth, a tight seal is crucial to stop bacteria from re-entering the root canal. This seal is made using gutta-percha and a sealer, creating a barrier that does not allow substances to pass through. However, newer bioceramic sealers and similar materials pose unique challenges for successful root canal therapy. These materials have two key characteristics: they are hydraulic, meaning they interact with fluids, and they react by producing calcium hydroxide that dissolves in solution [1, 5]. In addition, Bioceramics stick to the tooth's dentin through a process called alkaline etching, which happens due to the high alkaline nature of the sealer. This creates a mineral infiltration zone where the dentin and the sealer meet [6].

16.2   Introduction of the Case

Case of traumatic upper right maxillary central incisor with wide open apex and periapical radiolucency.

16.2.1   Patient Information

- Age: 22-year-old
- Gender: Female
- Medical history: Noncontributory

16.2.2   Tooth Information

16.2.2.1   Identification
Right maxillary central incisor (Tooth 11)

16.2.2.2   Dental History
Chief complaint: Patient reported with a chief complaint of intraoral swelling with tenderness on biting.

Clinical Examination Findings
Tooth 11 was tender to percussion. The buccal vestibule had intraoral swelling with tenderness on palpation.

Investigations
- Preoperative radiological assessment:
- The periapical radiograph revealed periapical radiolucency in relation to (irt) #11. The tooth had a wide open apex (Figure 16.1).

After the radiograph, CBCT was advised but the patient could not afford one, therefore it was decided to go ahead with radiographs and dental operating microscope (DOM) and then decide the course of the treatment plan.

Figure 16.1   Preoperative periapical radiograph showing wide open apex with periapical radiolucency.

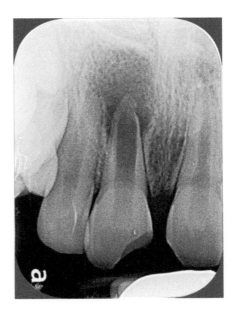

Sensibility Testing
1) Hot and cold test: No response
2) Electric pulp test (EPT): No response
3) Tenderness to percussion: Positive

16.2.2.3 Diagnosis (Pulpal and Periapical)

Necrotic pulp with symptomatic apical periodontitis (SAP)

16.2.2.4 Advice

- Root canal treatment with apical plug formation (apexification) with calcium silicate cement followed by obturation of the remaining root canal space
  OR
- Complete obturation of the root canal space with bioceramics.

16.3 Treatment Plan

The treatment was planned in different stages:

Stage 1
- Isolation of the tooth
- Gaining entry in the pulp chamber and locating the orifice
- Irrigating the canal
- Controlling bleeding
- Cleaning and disinfection of the root canal system
- Cleaning and shaping the canals (more of disinfection and less of shaping)
- Placement of calcium silicate cement amd formation of apical plug OR
- Complete obturation with bioceramics.

Stage 2
- Core buildup with suitable materials
- Postenedodontic full coverage restoration.

16.3.1 Treatment Procedure for the First Appointment

Buccal infiltration anesthesia was administered and the tooth was isolated with rubber dam isolation (Zirc, USA) (Figure 16.3). The endodontic access cavity was initiated under DOM (OPMI Pico, Carl Zeiss, Germany). Once the canal was located, it was irrigated with 3% sodium hypochlorite using IrriFlex needles (Produits Dentaires, Switzerland). The irrigation needle was chosen due to its flexible design and side vented portal of exits.

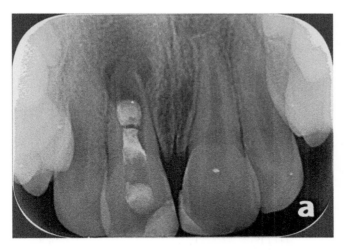

Figure 16.2 PA radiograph showing placement of MTA at the middle of the tooth length.

Ideally, there should have been a CBCT as there is evidence of apical resorption. Therefore, we are not very sure about the shape of the apical foramen. Since the patient could not afford CBCT, it was decided to visualize it clinically under the DOM and then plan for obturation.

Upon opening the canal, profuse bleeding was observed and attempt to arrest the bleeding was made using paper points dipped in hemolytic agents (Video 16.1). Once the bleeding was stopped, the periapical tissue could be clearly seen. The canal was dried with paper points and mineral trioxide aggregate (MTA) (Produits Dentaires, Switzerland) was placed at the level of the tissue. While placing MTA resistance could be felt while condensation, therefore, clinically it was felt that we were at the apex. Perapical radiograph was taken but the MTA was still at the middle of the canal (Figure 16.2). This meant either there was perforation resorption or the periapical tissue had ingressed from the apex.

It was decided to push the MTA to the radiographic length. In addition, since there was a perforating resorption suspected, it was decided to obturate the whole canal with calcium silicate cement and not use gutta-percha (GP) for obturation at any stage.

The MTA was pushed with the help of endodontic plugger and the entire canal was filled using incremental MTA technique (Video 16.2) where MTA is placed in increments and condensed using endodontic pluggers of suitable diameter (Figure 16.3). Immediate radiograph was taken to confirm the obturation with MTA (Figure 16.4).

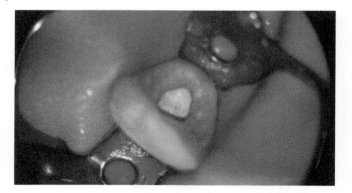

Figure 16.3 Complete obturation with MTA.

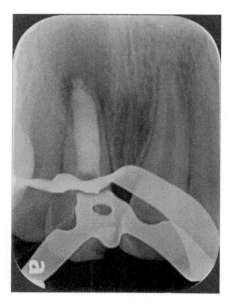

Figure 16.4 Radographic verification of complete obturation with MTA.

16.3.2 Treatment Procedure for the Second Appointment

The second appointment was planned to do the core buildup by placing Glass Ionomer cement (GIC) and then resin composite as the final restoration. It was confirmed on the radiograph (Figure 16.5).

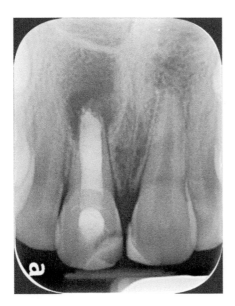

Figure 16.5 Radiographic verification of the obturation and the final restoration.

16.3.2.1 Irrigation Protocol

- 2.5% sodium hypochlorite throughout the cleaning and shaping procedure. Rinse with saline.
- 17% EDTA 1 ml/canal with sonic/ultrasonic activation. Rinse with saline.
- Final rinse with 2.5% sodium hypochlorite with internal heating with any instrument, e.g. Touch'n Heat, and sonic ultrasonic activation for 20–30 seconds per canal.

Flushing with saline between irrigants is a must, as it will stop the irrigants from reacting with each other.

Materials used for obturation: MTA for obturation, GIC, and resin composite for core buildup.

16.4 Technical Aspects

Traumatic injuries during tooth development can lead to failure in complete root development. In such cases, the root fails to achieve a natural constriction and we often see wide open apices accoumpanied with necrotic pulps. This is generally detected when the patient visits the dentist due to feeling tenderness on eating or intraoral swelling or sinus discharge in relation to those teeth. Wide open apex is seen in the PA which is then related to the traumatic injury few years back. Cone beam computed tomography (CBCT) *is a must in such cases.* However, in case CBCT is not feasible for some reason, DOM should be used to carefully examine the interior of the root canal space.

In case of resorptive defects, the perforating resorptions need to be closed with suitable bioactive materials.

In such cases where complete obturation with bioceramic is the treatment of choice, the following care should be taken:

- Minimal shaping of the root canals
- Maximum disinfection with recommended irrigation protocol
- Not pushing the irrigant beyond the apex in the periapical area
- Measuring the extent up to which endodontic plugger should go
- Placement of MTA at an adequate length
- Observing the radiographs and the root canal space for any signs of perforating resorptive areas
- Once MTA is set, fill the root canal space with thermoplasticized GP technique with gentle condensation.

Copious irrigation should be maintained throughout the procedure and endodontic files should not be used in dry canals.

16.5 Learning Objectives

The reader should be able to understand the following:

- The significance of proper reading of the preoperative radiograph
- Relating the radiographic findings with dental history of the patient
- The treatment plan to manage wide open apex cases
- The significance of sensibility testing to reach a proper diagnosis
- The role of irrigants for disinfecting the root canal system
- The choice of correct shaping technique in cases with weak root canal walls
- How to choose the correct material for obturation of the root canal space
- The technique, armamentarium required for bioceramic obturations
- The technique needed for filling the root canal space
- The concepts of understanding the prognosis of the tooth and trying to save the tooth instead of straight away extracting it.

16.6 Conclusion

Traumatic anterior teeth with wide open apex and resorptive defect can be suitably managed with apexification, closure of the resorptive defect, or complete obturation using the right kind of bioactive dental materials.

References

1 Camilleri, J. (2017). Will bioceramics be the future root canal filling materials? *Current Oral Health Reports* 4: 228–238.
2 Torabinejad, M. and Chivian, N. (1999). Clinical applications of mineral trioxide aggregate. *Journal of Endodontics* 25(3): 197–205.
3 Marciano, M.A., Costa, R.M., Camilleri, J. et al. (2014). Assessment of color stability of white mineral trioxide aggregate angelus and bismuth oxide in contact with tooth structure. *Journal of Endodontics* 40(8): 1235–1240.
4 Torabinejad, M., Hong, C., McDonald, F., and Ford, T.P. (1995). Physical and chemical properties of a new root-end filling material. *Journal of Endodontics* 21(7): 349–353.
5 Camilleri, J., Atmeh, A., Li, X., and Meschi, N. (2022). Present status and future directions: Hydraulic materials for endodontic use. *International Endodontic Journal* 55: 710–777.
6 Atmeh, A., Chong, E., Richard, G. et al. (2012). Dentin-cement interfacial interaction: calcium silicates and polyalkenoates. *Journal of Dental Research* 91(5): 454–459.

 To access the videos for this chapter, please go to

www.wiley.com/go/chopra/bioceramicsinendodontics

VIDEO 16.1 Attempts to arrest bleeding.
VIDEO 16.2 Obturation of the root canal with bioceramics.

17

Selective Management of a Case With Complicated Internal Morphology

Gergely Benyőcs[1] and Viresh Chopra[2,3,4]

[1] *Private Practitioner, Precedent Dental Office, Budapest, Hungary*
[2] *Adult Restorative Dentistry, Oman Dental College, Muscat, Oman*
[3] *Endodontology, Oman Dental College, Muscat, Oman*
[4] *Bart's London School of Medicine and Dentistry, Queen Mary University, London, UK*

CONTENTS

17.1 Introduction of the Case

Case of complicated internal morphology managed with selective primary root canal treatment approach using bioactive materials.

17.1.1 Patient Information

- Age: 38-year-old
- Gender: Female
- Medical history: Noncontributory

17.1.2 Tooth Information

17.1.2.1 Identification
Left maxillary lateral incisor (Tooth 22)

17.1.2.2 Dental History
Chief complaint: Patient reported with a chief complaint of moderate sensitivity around tooth 22.

Clinical Examination Findings
Tooth 11 was not mobile. Palpation was positive more buccally than palatally. Cold test was positive. Patient had normal general health conditions. Probing depth was within normal limits (Figure 17.1).

17.1.2.3 Investigations
- *Preoperative diagnostic assessment*
- *Preoperative radiological assessment*

Preoperative radiograph showed complex internal morphology of the tooth (Figure 17.2). Lateral radiolucency can be seen on the mesial aspect of the root.

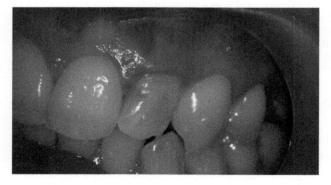

Figure 17.1 Clinical picture of tooth 22 showing discolored 22 and suspected mesial restoration.

Figure 17.2 Preoperative radiograph showing complex internal morphology irt 22.

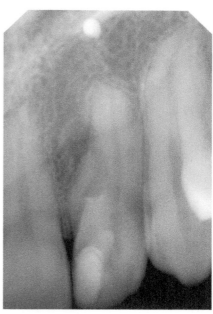

- *Cone Beam Computed Tomography*

  To confirm the complex internal morphology, cone beam computed tomography (CBCT) (CS 8100 3D, Carestream, Onex Corporation, Toronto, Ontario, Canada) was carried out (Figure 17.3).

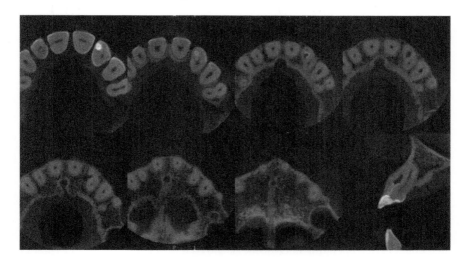

Figure 17.3 CBCT of tooth 22 showing dens invaginatus.

Sensibility Testing
1) Hot and cold test: Cold +ve but hot –ve
2) Electric pulp test (EPT): Delayed response
3) Tenderness to percussion: Positive

17.1.2.4 Diagnosis (Pulpal and Periapical)
Symptomatic apical periodontitis regarding indens, vital main root canal.

17.1.2.5 Advice
- Selective root canal treatment of only the indens root canal part and observe.
OR
- Complete root canal treatment of the root canal space.

Patient agreed to the selective root canal treatment approach, since it appeared to be a more conservative approach, and then keeping the tooth under watch.

17.2 Treatment Plan

The treatment was planned in two stages:

Stage 1
- Local anesthesia
- Isolation of the tooth
- Gaining entry in the pulp chamber and locating the orifice. (only the selected root canal space)
- Irrigating the canal
- Controlling bleeding, if any
- Cleaning and disinfection of the root canal system.
- Cleaning and shaping the canal
- Placement of intracanal medicament.

Stage 2
- Removal of intracanal medicament
- Finishing of the cleaning and shaping
- Obturation of the root canal

17.2.1 Treatment Procedure for the First Appointment

Buccal infiltration anesthesia was administered and the tooth was isolated with rubber dam isolation (Zirc, USA). The conservative endodontic access cavity was initiated under dental operating microscope (DOM) (OPMI Pico, Carl Zeiss, Germany). Once the indens canal was located (Figure 17.4), it was irrigated with 5.25% sodium hypochlorite using IrriFlex needles (Produits Dentaires, Switzerland). The irrigation needle was chosen due to its flexible design and side vented portal of exits.

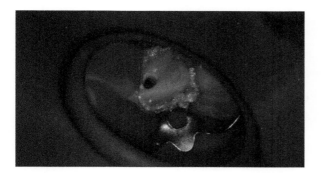

Figure 17.4 Conservative endodontic access cavity to locate the selected orifice (canal).

Stainless steel hand files were up to size 60 (Ready Steel FlexoFiles, Dentsply Maillefer, Germany), scouting before with 0.08 and 0.10 C-pilot files (VDW Gmbh, Germany). Once the canal was negotiated to full working length, intracanal medicament was placed. Calcium hydroxide paste (Calcipast, Cerkamed, Poland) was used between appointments. Patient became asymptomatic in two weeks.

17.2.2 Treatment Procedure for the Second Appointment

The second appointment was planned to remove the intracanal medicament. We cleannd and shaped, and obturated the root canal with gutta-percha and bioceramic root canal sealer (Totalfill BC Sealer – FKG Dentaire) (Figure 17.5). It was confirmed on the radiograph (Figure 17.6).

17.2.2.1 Irrigation Protocol

5.25% sodium hypochlorite was used for irrigation while shaping (Chlorax D 5.25%, Cerkamed, Poland) and 17% EDTA as a final rinse (EDTA solution Cerkamed, Poland) irrigation. Saline was used in-between irrigants and before obturation. Activation was carried out with ultrasonic device (NSK Varios 370), using IRRI 20 tip (Satelec Acteon). Flushing with saline between irrigants is a must as it will stop the irrigants from reacting with each other.

One month later, a glass fiber–resin reinforcement (everX Flow, GC, Europe) was carried out and a composite filling (Gradia Direct A3, GC, Japan).

Materials used for obturation: Gutta-percha and bioceramic sealer for obturation.

Control examinations were scheduled regularly. At the two-year follow-up, the patient was asymptomatic. Examination was negative. Cold test was positive. Postoperative radiograph showed satisfactory healing of the lateral radiolucent lesion (Figure 17.7).

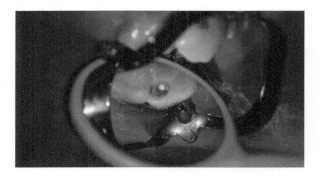

Figure 17.5 Obturation of the indens root canal.

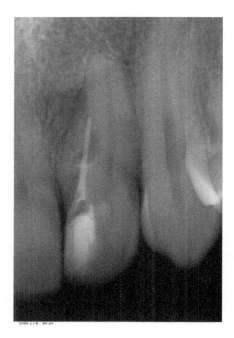

Figure 17.6 Radiographic verification of the obturation.

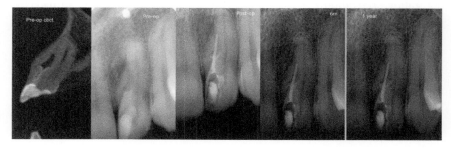

Figure 17.7 Radiograhic flow showing the progress of selective root canal treatment resulting in healing of the lesion.

17.3   Technical Aspects

Complex internal morphologies of the teeth might not be a routine in endodontic practice, but they do appear every now and then. Initially, these variations can be detected on preoperative radiograph. However, CBCT is a must in such cases to confirm the radiographic observation and decide the treatment protocol as per the observations. In case of resorptive defects, the perforating resorptions need to be closed with suitable bioactive materials.

In such cases selective root canal treatment can be a new approach as the clinician is trying to treat the infected part only. In cases where root canals are not connected with each other, selective conservative treatment can be done and the teeth can be kept under observation and complete root canal treatment of all the canals can be done in case the initial treatment does not show a positive response. However, more research needs to be done with this approach and substantial evidence needs to be present in the literature. The clinician should know the following:

- Use the latest technology for diagnosis
- Minimal shaping of the root canals
- Maximum disinfection with recommended irrigation protocol
- Not pushing the irrigant beyond the apex in the periapical area
- Use of bioactive materials does get an edge over conventional materials.
- Observe the radiographs and the root canal space for any signs of perforating resorptive areas.

Copious irrigation should be maintained throughout the procedure and endodontic files should not be used in dry canals.

17.4   Learning Objectives

The reader should be able to understand the following:

- The significance of proper reading of the preoperative radiograph.
- Relating the radiographic findings with the dental history of the patient.
- Significance of CBCT for diagnosis of such cases.
- The treatment plan to manage dens invaginatus.
- How to plan selective root canal treatment approach.
- The role of irrigants for disinfecting the root canal system.
- The choice of correct shaping technique in cases with weak root canal walls.
- How to choose the correct material for obturation of the root canal space.
- The technique, armamentarium required for bioceramic obturations.
- The technique needed for filling the root canal space.
- The concepts of understanding the prognosis of the tooth and trying to save the tooth instead of straight away extracting it.

17.5 Conclusion

Variations in internal morphology need to be properly investigated to reach a definitive diagnosis. Use of CBCT is a must in such cases as it not only helps to confirm the initial preoperative radiographic observations, but also helps to plan the treatment protocol, especially if the clinician is wishing to perform selective root canal treatment.

18

Retreatment of a Maxillary Molar With Complex Internal Morphology

Gergely Benyőcs[1] and Viresh Chopra[2,3,4]

[1] *Private Practitioner, Precedent Dental Office, Budapest, Hungary*
[2] *Adult Restorative Dentistry, Oman Dental College, Muscat, Oman*
[3] *Endodontology, Oman Dental College, Muscat, Oman*
[4] *Bart's London School of Medicine and Dentistry, Queen Mary University, London, UK*

CONTENTS

18.1   Introduction of the Case

Case of retreatment in a maxillary molar with six root canal orifices but four apical exits.

18.2   Patient Information

- Age: 43-year-old
- Gender: Male
- Medical history: Noncontributory

18.2.1   Tooth Information

18.2.1.1   Identification
Left maxillary first molar (Tooth 26)

18.2.1.2   Dental History
- Chief complaint: Patient reported with a chief complaint of moderate, diffuse pain on the left side.
- Clinical examination findings:
  Periodontal probing depth was within normal limits; tooth was slightly movable. Palpation was positive more buccally than lingually.

18.2.1.3   Investigations
- Preoperative diagnostic assessment
- Preoperative radiological assessment

Preoperative PA radiograph showed previous root canal treatment with periapical radiolucency. The orthopantomogram (OPG) showed multiple root canals present in the oral cavity. The obturation is suspected to be short in the buccal canals (Figure 18.1).

18.2.1.4   Diagnosis (Pulpal and Periapical)
Failed previous root canal treatment with symptomatic apical periodontitis.

18.2.1.5   Advice
Retreatment of the previous root canal treatment.

18.3   Treatment Plan

The treatment was planned in two stages:

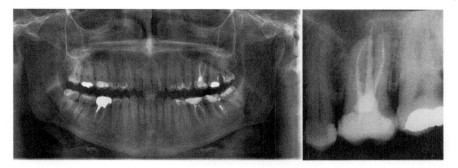

Figure 18.1 Preoperative PA and OPG showing previous root canal treatment in tooth 26. Periapical radiolucency can be seen in both the radiographs.

Stage 1
- Local anesthesia
- Isolation of the tooth
- Gaining entry in the pulp chamber and locating the previous gutta-percha
- Removal of the previous obturating material
- Irrigating the located canals
- Explore the access cavity for missing canals in the initial treatment
- Working length determination
- Initial negotiation and disinfection of the root canal system
- Placement of intracanal medicament.

Stage 2
- Removal of intracanal medicament
- Final of the cleaning and shaping
- Obturation of the root canal system.

18.3.1 Treatment Procedure for the First Appointment

Buccal infiltration anesthesia was administered; the tooth was isolated with rubber dam isolation and the tooth was seen under the microscope preoperatively (Figure 18.2).

Endodontic access was prepared using an Endo Access bur. The previous GP was located. The coronal part of the GP in the pulp chamber was removed with ultrasonic scaler. Old obturation material was removed with Reciproc Blue R-25. (VDW Gmbh, Germany). Drainage of pus could be seen upon removing the GPs. Irrigation was performed using sodium hypochlorite and saline alternatively (Figure 18.3).

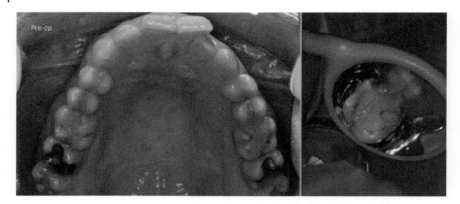

Figure 18.2   Clinical picture showing preoperative condition of 26 and rubber dam isolation of 26.

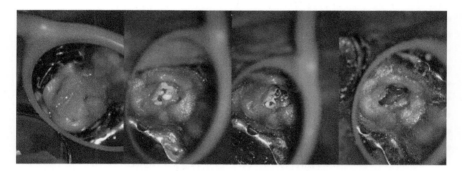

Figure 18.3   Stages of retreatment from preoperative, location of GPs, removal of GPs and location of initial canals.

Root canals were scouted with 0.08 and 0.10 C-pilot files (VDW Gmbh, Germany). Working length was determined electronically. Intracanal medicament was placed and patient recalled for second appointment. Calcium hydroxide paste (Calcipast, Cerkamed, Poland) was used as intracanal medicament.

18.3.2   Treatment Procedure for the Second Appointment

Intracanal medicament was removed using irrigants and rotary files. Endodontic access cavity was explored for any extra canal orifices.

On careful exploration, 06 orifices were found and clinical verified as root canals (Figure 18.4).

Cleaning and shaping were completed with Race 20/02 (FKG Dentaire) regarding to MB2 and MB3. MB1, P and DB, DB1 root canals were shaped up to Reciproc

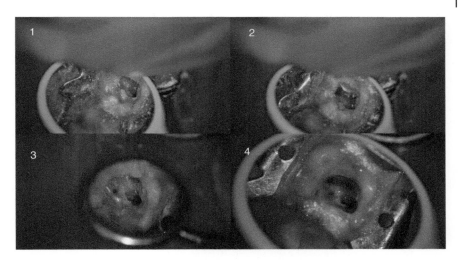

Figure 18.4 Clinical pictures showing stages of exploration of access cavity and canal orifice location. (1) Modified access cavity. (2) GP removal in process. (3) Location of extra canal orifices. (4) Modifies access cavity with all the previously missed root canal orifices.

Blue R-50. (VDW Gmbh, Germany). After cleaning and shaping master cones were verified and the canals prepared for obturation. The canals were left moist for bioceramic sealer to be used along GP as the core obturating material. Obturation was performed using GP and tricalcium silicate–based sealer (TotalFill BC Sealer – FKG Dentaire).

All the canal orifices were obturated (6 orifices) and verified clinically as well as radiographically (Figure 18.5).

Materials used for obturation: GP and bioceramic sealer for obturation.

The recall radiographs showed efficient healing in the periapical area and, clinically, the patient became asymptomatic (Figure 18.6).

Clinical picture showed 6 canal orifices. However, MB3 and MB2 were meeting in the apical area, hence one portal of exit (Figure 18.7).

18.3.2.1 Irrigation Protocol

5.25% sodium hypochlorite was used for irrigation while shaping (Chlorax D 5.25%, Cerkamed, Poland) and 17% EDTA as a final rinse (Edta Solution Cerkamed, Poland irrigation). Saline was used between irrigants and before obturation. Activation was carried out with ultrasonic device (NSK Varios 370) using IRRI 20 tip (Satelec Acteon). Flushing with saline between irrigants is a must as it will stop the irrigants from reacting with each other.

One month later, a glass fiber resin reinforcement (everX Flow, GC, Europe) was carried out and a composite filling (Gradia Direct A3, GC, Japan.)

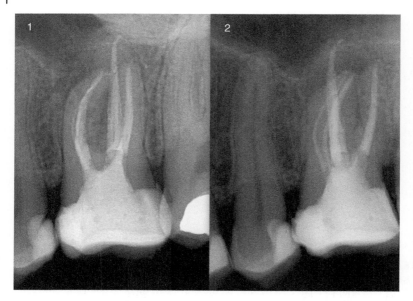

Figure 18.5 Postoperative radiographs showing obturation of the complete root canal system. (1) Post obturation radiograph. (2) Mesial angulation radiograph showing 5 root canals and 4 portals of exit.

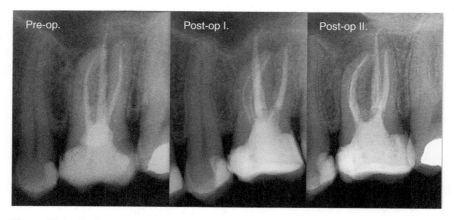

Figure 18.6 Radiographs comparing initial situation with immediate postoperative and 6-month follow-up showing satisfactory healing.

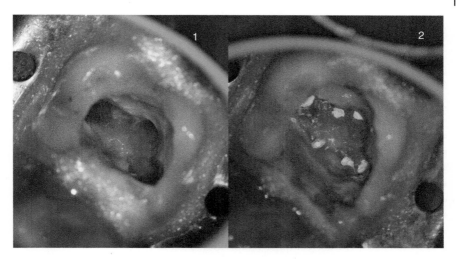

Figure 18.7 (1) Clinical picture showing the 06 located root canal orifices after cleaning and shaping. (2) Clinical picture showing the 06 located root canal orifices after obturation.

18.4 Technical Aspects

Missed canal is one of the main reasons resulting in failure of the primary root canal treatment. Careful examination of the preoperative radiograph and clinical access cavity leads to location of all the canal orifices present. Missing any one of them results in inadequate cleaning and disinfection of the root canal system. Leftover biological tissue can easily lead to failure of the root canal treatment by causing apical periodontist or periapical abscess. Nonsurgical retreatment is the treatment of choice in such cases. *CBCT can be helpful in such cases, however, if the endodontic treatment/retreatment is performed under DOM, then such cases can be solved efficiently without a CBCT too.*

The clinician should be well aware about the following:

- Reading a preoperative radiograph
- Modifying the access cavity as per the case
- Locating all the canal orifices
- Maximum disinfection with recommended irrigation protocol
- Not pushing the irrigant beyond the apex in the periapical area
- Use of bioactive materials does give an edge over conventional materials.

Copious irrigation should be maintained throughout the procedure and endodontic files should not be used in dry canals.

18.5 Learning Objectives

The reader should be able to understand the following:

- The significance of proper reading of the preoperative radiograph.
- Relating the radiographic findings with dental history of the patient.
- Significance of CBCT for diagnosis of such cases.
- The treatment plan to manage dens invaginatus.
- How to plan selective root canal treatment approach.
- The role of irrigants for disinfecting the root canal system.
- The choice of correct shaping technique in cases with weak root canal walls.
- How to choose the correct material for obturation of the root canal space.
- The technique, armamentarium required for bioceramic obturations.
- The technique needed for filling the root canal space.
- The concepts of understanding the prognosis of the tooth and trying to save the tooth instead of straight away extracting it.

18.6 Conclusion

Retreatment protocols are different and more complex than primary root canal treatment protocols. The clinician should be well-versed with the available options for retreatment files and latest biomaterials present that can be used for efficient results.

Index

Note: page numbers in *italics* refer to figures; those in **bold** to tables.

Bioceramics in Endodontics, First Edition. Edited by Viresh Chopra.
© 2024 John Wiley & Sons, Inc. Published 2024 by John Wiley & Sons, Inc.
Companion website: www.wiley.com/go/chopra/bioceramicsinendodontics